THE
GREEN WITCH

THE GREEN WITCH
A MODERN WOMAN'S HERBAL

BARBARA GRIGGS

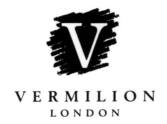

VERMILION
LONDON

For Ninka

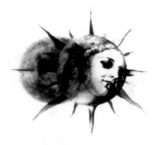

First published in 1993

3 5 7 9 10 8 6 4

First published in the United Kingdom in 1993 by Vermilion
an imprint of Ebury Press
Random House, 20 Vauxhall Bridge Road, London SW1V 2SA

Random House Australia (Pty) Limited
20 Alfred Street, Milsons Point, Sydney,
New South Wales 2061, Australia

Random House New Zealand Limited
18 Poland Road, Glenfield,
Auckland 10, New Zealand

Random House South Africa (Pty) Limited
PO Box 337, Bergvlei, 2012 South Africa

Random House UK Limited Reg. No. 954009

A CIP catalogue record for this book
is available from the British Library

ISBN 0-7126-4725-2

Text design by Sara Kidd
Edited by Pamela Dix

Papers used by Ebury Press are natural recyclable products made from wood
grown in sustainable forests. In addition the paper in this book is acid free.

Typeset by SX Composing Limited, Rayleigh, Essex
Printed and bound in Great Britain by Clays Ltd., St Ives plc

This book gives non-specific, general advice and should not be relied on
as a substitute for proper medical consultation. The author and publisher
cannot accept responsibility for illness arising out of the failure to seek
medical advice from a doctor.

CONTENTS

———o———

Foreword   6

FOREWORD

On a warm summer evening many years ago, I sat talking to friends in their fragrant garden. My hostess and I both had small babies, and we chatted happily about them, swopping experiences, ideas, suggestions. We talked, too, of their health. But here I found that my own worries about childhood ailments – colic, colds, sleeplessness – were not shared by my hostess. 'You see,' she remarked idly, 'my mother is a herbalist, and my bathroom cabinet is full of wonderful herbal remedies.'

A herbalist for a mother? A cupboard full of herbal remedies? I had never heard of such a thing. It was the early 1970s, and in my occasional forays into the funny little health-food shops of the time, I had noticed packets of medicinal teas, bottles of herbal cough mixtures, jars of ointments with unfamiliar names. I had always assumed, though, that these were little more than faded souvenirs of the past, like the bowls of pot-pourri I could remember sniffing curiously in houses I had visited as a child. That herbalists still existed, and that one of my own friends believed in the efficacy of such out-dated remedies – these were new ideas to me.

That conversation launched me into a lifetime voyage of discovery. Herbal medicine has a history almost as old as humanity; it became my study to trace and document that history, a study of 20 years so far! As I learned more, and met more experts from this extraordinary world, I began applying my new expertise to my own domestic needs.

Our children grew up resigned to the fact that while their friends were given little white pills when they were ill, they themselves would be gagging over doses of strange, dark brown liquids; that instead of sugary pink medicines, they would be sipping cupfuls of odd-tasting herbal tea; and that their coughs and colds would be treated with pungent oils rubbed into their chests, with old-fashioned Mustard footbaths, and with teaspoons of a lethal mixture based on Cayenne that burned all the way down their throats. 'Mamma's *wonderful* herbal remedies' became a wry if affectionate family joke – but they worked.

Very slowly I began to acquire just a little of the knowledge that would have been elementary to millions of women in the past.

Through the ages, in almost every corner of the globe, the woman of the house has been a herbal expert by necessity. There was no other medicine available, and often no practitioner except herself. She picked up a rough working knowledge of the available medicinal plants from her own mother, from friends, from local tradition, perhaps from a visiting shaman or wise woman. Gradually she accumulated her own store of skilled knowledge, to be transmitted in turn to her own daughters.

The plant world supplied her with far more than medicine, however. From the plants that grew locally, almost all her household needs had to be met: much of the food and drink her family consumed; the yarns she wove into cloth for the family wardrobe, or ropes, mats and hangings; the rudimentary cleaning materials and insect-repellants she used for her home or for family hygiene; the skin and hair-care products she devised to beautify herself and her daughters. Harvesting and processing the plant material to produce all this can have left her with little or no leisure time.

It is hard today to imagine such a world. Our lives have been revolutionized by modern technology and the invention of synthetic chemicals, and they have certainly been made far easier. A trip to the supermarket or High Street chemist will supply us with foodstuffs from all over the world, much of which will keep for days, weeks or even months; with household cleaners, detergents, disinfectants and polishes; with shampoos, bath-oils, hair dyes, skin-care products and cosmetics; and with a wide range of ready-made medicines.

An Elizabethan housewife would surely have been green with envy if transported to a modern High Street supermarket – and I would not want to change places with her.

Yet the conviction that we are the lucky ones began fading some time ago. More and more of us today are rediscovering the Green wisdom that was thrown out as old wives' tales generations back. Those old wives, we are finding out, knew a thing or two well worth the learning.

I have rediscovered the pleasure as well as the good sense of fresh food eaten in its own season. I have learned that herbs and spices not only enhance the taste of food but can influence our health in many important ways. I have also re-learned a truth familiar to every Medieval housewife – that the most delicious food can be the very best medicine.

For a wide range of the common ailments normally treated at home – toothache; upset stomach; grazes; insomnia; earache; burns and scalds; sore throat; bouts of diarrhoea; 'flu; odd bugs; mild viral infection; coughs and colds; and chills – herbal remedies are more effective and certainly cheaper than those you buy at the chemist. In fact they are often to hand in my own kitchen. Even when the doctor is called on to treat more serious illnesses, there are always mild and safe herbal remedies which can relieve the more distressing symptoms and hasten recovery. And at times of real stress, or when my workload is particularly heavy, I

turn to the herbal world for the marvellous tonics which keep me going.

Like millions of women, too, I've noticed that skin creams, tonics and lotions made from natural ingredients such as Jojoba, Cucumber, Avocado and Elderflower seem kinder to, and feel better on, my skin than the synthetic chemicals used in modern skin-care products. A few drops of essential oil in the bath can be soothing, relaxing or tonic to my spirits the way strong-smelling, bought bubble-baths never are.

I am not sprinkling rushes or strewing herbs around my home yet, but when I need a pleasant room-freshener after a party, an effective domestic disinfectant, or good moth-repellant, essential oils supply these too.

Along my journey of discovery I have acquired a new respect for the marvellous Green world of plants and their incredible versatility.

Much of what I have learned is quite ancient. They knew all about the magical prowess of Garlic when the Pyramids were built. Onions, Ginger and Ginseng all feature in the earliest known medical manuscript. Three hundred years before Christ, Hippocrates was recommending Barley water for convalescents. Much of what any modern herbalist knows about common European medicinal plants was recorded nearly 2000 years ago, in the first Western Herbal, written by a military surgeon in Nero's armies called Dioscorides.

I have been lucky enough to have had brilliant teachers. Some of them were practising herbalists, naturopaths, aromatherapists, who generously allowed me to draw on their stores of knowledge and experience. Some were my readers, who wrote with suggestions and information, as well as questions, after reading one of my articles in *Country Living*. Some were members of audiences when I have given talks on herbal medicine; I often learned as much as I taught on these occasions. At one such, when I had listed my favourite medicinal herbs, a group of Asian women came up to me afterwards and asked how I could have failed to mention Turmeric; it is as widely used in Indian domestic medicine as aspirin is in Britain, they told me. I scribbled notes for the next half hour while they explained eagerly what a marvellous and versatile medicine Turmeric is. I no longer think of it as the poor man's Saffron.

Many more of my teachers were unknown to me personally, the authors of books which I have on my own shelves (some almost worn out by continuous reference), or pored over in great libraries; or of articles I read in magazines or newspapers. I hope that *The Green Witch* will become one of *your* essential reference books, and that you will explore its pages over and over again for the fascinating remedies and recipes that I love to use.

There is no such thing as a 'new' herb, but over the last decades particularly, dozens more useful and important herbs have been added to our repertory in the West. Some we have learned of from other countries and other cultures, such as Guarana, the great anti-stress tonic from the Amazon; others are native herbs whose marvellous curative powers are discovered by serendipity and confirmed in sober hospital settings, like Feverfew, the migraine remedy. Another important newcomer is Evening Primrose, the first identified plant-source of a vital essential oil, gamma-linolenic acid.

Other welcome additions to my personal Receipt book are the marvellous essential oils now available. Among my favourites: antiseptic Tea Tree, all-purpose Lavender, Geranium – the lovely stimulant and anti-depressant, and

Eucalyptus, wonderful for the respiratory tract.

Almost nothing in this book is original. The most I can claim is to be an eager apprentice of an art many thousands of years old: and I'm still learning.

I hope that you too will profit from this wonderful Green Witchcraft.

CAUTION Throughout this book, herbs are recommended as food, made up into drinks, or in remedies for particular health problems. The herbs mentioned are of little or no known toxicity; in the quantities or doses suggested, they are perfectly safe for general consumption. Where caution is advisable, I have noted the fact. Just occasionally, however, a herb can provoke an unexpected reaction in an individual – and not all herbal remedies will work for everyone alike.

When harvesting herbs growing wild – for instance, Hawthorn blossom, Plantain or Chickweed – be absolutely sure of your identification. If necessary, use one of the many excellent illustrated guides.

Essential oils should always be used with the greatest possible care and never used neat on the skin, unless otherwise suggested by a professional practitioner. Women who are pregnant, or who are trying to be, should avoid taking herbal remedies by mouth, except under the direction of a qualified herbalist; they should be careful even with common herbal teas such as Peppermint, and other herbs of the aromatic *Labiatae* family – Sage, Rosemary, Thyme and others.

A good cook is half a physician.
Nicholas Culpeper

HOME
and
KITCHEN

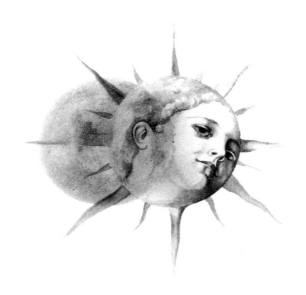

HERBS AROUND THE HOME

In the Middle Ages, herbs and flowers were prized as much for their aroma as for their good looks. This is not surprising, as the Medieval home or castle was a malodorous place by our standards, given the lack of running water, flushing lavatories, and refrigeration which we take for granted. To conceal the unpleasant odours, the Medieval housewife strewed sweet-smelling herbs on the floor which gave off an agreeable smell when crushed underfoot; she hung bunches of aromatic herbs in the kitchen, larder and linen-cupboard; and buried her nose in bunches of fragrant herbs for a treat. If she was lucky enough to have a tiny walled flower-garden, she filled it with the sweetest-smelling flowers, to escape into whenever she could.

Herbs were also relied on to help keep under control the armies of fleas, lice, cockroaches, moths, rodents and other domestic pests that were an ever-present part of Medieval life.

The modern housewife does not use herbs for these purposes. She buys aerosol cans filled with powerful chemicals to slaughter unwanted insect life. If the dog or cat has brought fleas home, a collar impregnated with powerful chemicals is fastened around their neck. If she is fastidious about smells, she may spray her lavatory with a chemically perfumed room-freshener. And now that herbs are modish, she can fill a bowl with one of those packets of 'pot-pourri' now being sold in supermarkets. I find the powerful synthetic smell of these room-fresheners and mass-produced pot-pourris nauseating, and would not have them in my home at any price.

Insect-repellants and room fresheners are just two of the domestic needs once served by herbs, now catered for by synthetic chemicals. The lengthening list of those we scatter so liberally round our homes today – cleaners, detergents, shampoos and polishes – are a form of pollution which can have a very negative effect on our health. They can lower our resistance and make us more liable to allergic problems such as eczema and hay-fever; the incidence of both is increasing dramatically.

Among the cocktail of chemicals commonly found in homes and offices in the 1990s are those used in construction, fireproofing, insulation materials and others used to treat wood and carpets. Insulation, central heating and air-conditioning in office buildings can send the circulating levels of such polluting chemicals rocketing. There are those whose homes are literally making them ill; Sick Building Syndrome is a reality which is now taken very seriously indeed.

Fortunately, there is an alternative to the man-made chemical option in our own homes: herbs and green plants, which are often just as effective, smell a great deal nicer, and perform their tasks without risk to our health or that of the environment. Many of these useful plants – among them insect-repellants, disinfectants and room fresheners – were familiar household aids centuries ago. Today we can rediscover their usefulness.

Modern scientific research is also rapidly establishing an entirely new role for plants: that of countering the chemical pollution of the modern environment, from homes and offices to public buildings such as hospitals and airports. Some forms of noise pollution are yielding to Green power, too.

It is now being shown that green plants can help counter stress. The very colour green has long been acknowledged as restful to our eyes; the traditional 'green room' provided in theatres since 1687 was there to relieve actors' eyes from the glare of the limelight. In one fascinating study, it was shown that hospital patients got better faster when their rooms had a view of trees and plants than when they looked out only at other buildings. The firm Rentokil is sponsoring research designed to test and confirm the benefits of green plants in the workplace, looking at areas such as reduced absenteeism and lower stress levels.

Use the following pages to see just how you can protect, clean and freshen your living environment through the natural, Green world.

Plants Against Pollution

If America sends a manned space-station up into orbit, it will be decorated with green plants. This will not be simply to make life more homely up among the stars; the plants will have a specific function: to counter pollution in the space-station by over 100 toxic chemicals.

Research into the detoxifying powers of plants began in the US NASA laboratories in the 1970s, when it became clear that such pollution could be a major problem in the air-conditioned closed-system space station. NASA's then chief scientist, Dr Bill Wolverton, proposed that since plants could recycle oxygen, they might also be able to recycle pollutants.

In intriguing experiments carried out by NASA over several years, plants were placed in sealed plexiglass containers, into which polluting, chemical-laden gases were pumped. To the scientists' astonishment, a number of plants – mainly tropical – turned out to be marvellous anti-pollution agents; they actually absorbed the dangerous chemicals into stem, root or leaf, transforming them into useful plant nutrients.

Among the most worrying of the chemicals that turn up in homes and offices these days are benzene, TCE or trichloroethylene, and formaldehyde. The plants tested absorbed varying quantities of all three chemicals. Low levels of chemicals were absorbed by the leaves alone; much more was extracted when air was filtered through the plant roots, surrounded by soil containing activated carbon.

Dr Wolverton has been continuing the research ever since – he now works for a private company. At least one British company, Green Scene, has put it to practical use, supplying similar plant systems for public buildings, offices and – more recently – homes.

High levels of chemicals are more likely to be found in big modern office-blocks than homes, but benzene, TCE and formaldehyde can turn up even in your own sitting-room. Much the worst of these is benzene, which can irritate the skin and eye, cause nausea, giddiness and headaches, loss of appetite and drowsiness. Exposure even to low levels of benzene can eventually cause nervous problems and anaemia. Benzene is found in tobacco smoke, synthetic fibres, plastics, inks and detergents.

TCE turns up in dry-cleaning materials, paints and varnishes, lacquers, adhesives, wood-finishes, and photocopiers – now standard equipment in offices. The American National Institute of Cancer Research claimed in 1975 that TCE could be responsible for cancer of the liver.

New carpeting, wall coverings, fibreboard, plywood, resins, and natural gas are among common sources of formaldehyde, which can irritate the mucous membranes of the mouth, eyes and throat, make life worse for asthma sufferers and even cause throat cancer.

It would be hard to throw out all these chemicals, even if we wanted to.

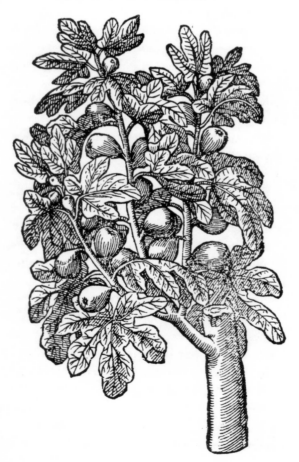

Here again, though, plants can come to man's rescue. Most green plants will recycle some pollutants; the following have been shown to be particularly effective. When you are choosing plants to have around the home, it makes sense to consider these. And what nicer or healthier present for a patient in one of our polluted hospitals?

Spider plants (*Chlorophytum elatum*) and Heart Leaf Philodendron (*Philodendron oxycardium*) are both effective at removing formaldehyde. Also effective in this respect are: Azaleas (*Rhododendron indicum*); that tall inflexible plant Mother-in-Law's Tongue (*Sanseveria laurentii*); Poinsettias (*Euphorbia pulcherrima*), and Fig trees (*Ficus moraceae*).

Those plants most effective against benzene were English Ivy (*Hedera helix*); Marginata (*Dracaena marginata*) – an attractive spiky plant; and Golden Pothos (*Scindapsus aureus*).

The lovely Peace Lily (*Spathiphyllum 'Mauna Loa')*, with its shiny green leaves and elegant white blooms, won first prize for helping clear TCE, followed by the attractive Dragon Tree (*Dracaena deremensis* 'Janet Craig' and 'Warnecker').

There is even a very spiky-looking cactus – *Cereus peruvianus* – which is said to eat up electro-magnetic pollution when placed on top of your computer or television. Its native habitat is the high plateaux of Mexico, where the sun's radiation is very intense; Swiss scientists speculated that it should be able to absorb high levels of electro-magnetic radiation. Environmental consultant Peter Campbell, who has supplied numbers of these plants to his customers, found this confirmed by muscle testing; he points out, though, that there is not as yet any acknowledged scientific test to measure this suggested effect. There are many satisfied customers, however, who claim to have diminished adverse effects – headaches, fatigue and blurred vision for example.

It is probable that other plants, as yet un-studied, have the same ability to soak up un-wanted pollutants from our environment. **N.B.** a number of the most popular house-plants can be toxic, or irritating to the skin; among them are: Amaryllis; Poinsettia; Ivy; Hyacinth; Swiss cheese plants; Chrysanthe-mum leaves. Enjoy your plants – but do not fondle or eat them!

INSECT-REPELLANTS

The fragrant herbs strewn on the floor in homes for centuries were not just a pretty smell. They had a practical purpose too: that of repelling fleas, flies and other household pests. If you do not like the chemical reek of modern pest-control sprays, or worry about their en-vironmental effect, try a Green solution – you may find it just as effective.

KITCHEN PESTS

Strings of Garlic and bundles of Chilli peppers hung from the rafters of an old-fashioned kitchen have more than eye-appeal; flies and other pests do not care for them. Pots of aromatic plants – Sage, Thyme, Origan, Basil – growing on your window-sill will deter them too, and help keep your kitchen clean and sweet-smelling.

Rue – that fast-growing little bushy plant with leaves that are tinged blue and smell oddly when rubbed between the fingers – has always been considered powerful protection against fleas, flies and noxious insects. Try keeping a small pot on your kitchen window-sill in the summer. Mint is reputed to be dis-agreeable to flies too.

Italian butchers always tuck sprigs of Rose-mary between their joints of pork. It is a sound practice; aromatic herbs help counter microbial activity in meat, poultry, game and fish. If I buy these food-stuffs, I tuck sprigs of fresh herbs – Thyme, Bayleaves, Sage, Rosemary, Marjoram, and a Garlic clove or two – inside or under them before I store them loosely wrapped in paper in the fridge. If I do not have fresh herbs, I sprinkle them with one of the wonderful mixtures of culinary herbs you can buy these days. These herbs will not only make meat, poultry or fish safer to eat, they will flavour the food too.

If you rent a house or apartment in the Mediterranean in summer, you may find your kitchen overrun by ants every time you leave

---

Towards the end of Madame Errazuriz's many years in France, her favourite great niece, Madame Lopez-Wilshaw, went to stay with her in the house at Biarritz and described the old lady (with hair like white silk that she washed in rain water) wandering barefoot among the rosemary bushes and the lavender in her garden. 'Everything in Aunt Eugenia's house smelled so good, everything was so clean,' she said. 'The bathrooms had such wonderful soap, and lots of rose-geranium salts. The towels were thick, heavy ones with fringes, and smelled of lavender. It was so peaceful to be with her, almost the peace of a convent. She was such a simple human being. Everything in her life had quality and simplicity. . . .'

(Cecil Beaton, 1954)
The Glass of Fashion

---

even a crumb of food out. Track down their point of entry into the house, and sprinkle plenty of Cayenne pepper around it.

A couple of Bayleaves tucked into jars of rice, flour, cereals or pulses will help deter weevils.

FLEAS

When I was working on the last chapters of *Green Pharmacy*, my history of herbal medicine, I escaped from my family for 10 days to a flat in Amsterdam for some intensive work. Alas, the flat turned out to be alive with fleas, from neighbouring cats upstairs and down. The fleas jumped merrily around my notes spread out on the carpet, and feasted on me in bed at night. The chemical solution – fumigating the place with fierce chemicals, and leaving it locked up for a few hours – was not on, as I could not spare the time.

In desperation, I consulted one of my herbals, and read that Southernwood – *Artemisia abrotanum* – was an excellent flea-repellent. I tracked down a herbalist, bought up their entire supply, and scattered it freely all over the floor and under the sheets on my bed. I never saw another flea.

Southernwood contains a strongly smelling volatile oil similar to that of Wormwood. Moths do not like it any more than fleas do, for which reason the French have christened the plant *Garderobe*.

If your dog or cat is flea-infested, tie a shoestring dipped in Eucalyptus or Cypress oil round their neck for a few hours; put fresh Walnut leaves in their baskets or beds – no insect will touch these; or Eucalyptus leaves; or a sprig or two of fresh Pennyroyal, one of the Mint family. The Latin name of this plant – *Mentha pulegium* – is a reminder of this particular usefulness: *pulex* is Latin for flea. These little creatures can migrate from pets to become a nuisance to human beings too; if so, put plenty of Pennyroyal, dried or fresh, around the house; leave it as long as possible before sweeping it up.

John A. Rohrbach, a vet from Perth who uses herbal treatment for his animals, lists a number of other herbs that fleas do not care for: Wormwood; Feverfew; Camphor Plant; Catmint; Tansy; Lavender; Rosemary; and Sage. In summertime, he suggests, scatter the leaves and flowers in the house, patio, or garden; in winter use them dried. As extra protection, make an infusion of 1 level teaspoon of any of these herbs in a cupful of boiling water. When cool, sprinkle it lightly on your dog's coat before taking him out for a walk.

To fumigate a room infested with fleas or other pests, Juliette de Baïracli Levy suggests the following. Sprinkle a tablespoon of Cayenne pepper on a tin lid; place it over a low flame (use a nightlight in a jar) and seal up the room while the acrid fumes fill it. It is safe for human beings after the room has been well aired!

You can also fill a plant-mister with water and a few drops of an insect-repellent Aromatic oil – Eucalyptus is particularly effective – and spray it round odd corners where fleas are likely to lurk.

MOSQUITOES

Mosquito bites are maddeningly, painfully irritating (see p.151 for remedies). If you get enough of them, the accumulating poison in your system can make you feel ill and wretched. If you are as susceptible as I am, and in mosquito territory, the best form of repellent is total cover-up. (In tropical countries, where a single mosquito bite could spell malaria or other diseases, total cover-up as far as possible is mandatory.)

If you are less susceptible, or the mosquitoes

less numerous, then you can depend on an effective insect-repellent and go around with bare arms and legs like a normal human being.

The chemical used in most mosquito-repellants – Diethyltoluamide (DEET) is quite powerful; the use of these repellants over long periods – particularly for babies or very small children – does not seem like a good idea. Some of the most effective (jungle-tested) new mosquito-repellents on the market, however, are made with a lower doses of DEET, boosted with one or another of the aromatic essential oils known to be useful insect-repellents. There are a number of mosquito-repellents now available that are pure aromatherapy.

You can also make your own repellants, experimenting to find the combination which most successfully repels them without irritating your own nose too much. (High doses of these oils, unfortunately, can be disagreeable to humans too.)

Choose from Eucalyptus, Cloves, Geranium, Onion, Peppermint, Rosemary and Citronella. Pick 2 or 3, and add them to some Almond or Soya oil in the proportions of 4 drops to a teaspoonful; apply the oil to exposed skin. Geranium has not only a lovely smell – one of my own great favourites – but is particularly effective.

US health-writer Lelord Kordel swears by a strong infusion of Feverfew, both leaves and flowers, sponged on the skin and allowed to dry. He has used it since he was a boy, he says, and has never found an insect-repellant more effective.

Amsterdammers put huge pots of the species of Geranium that produces Citronella oil at their open windows in summer; these seem to be very successful in keeping out the mosquitoes that haunt the canals. Citronella candles, which you can buy at some herbal

suppliers, are also strikingly effective.

A few drops of these oils can be added to a saucer of water, or put on an essential-oil burner, for further discouragement.

Another smell that mosquitoes dislike is Onion. During summer holidays in the south of Spain, when the children were small and mosquito netting was unobtainable locally, I used to cut up huge Onions and leave them on the window-sill and by the girls' beds – to their strenuous protests!

To clear terraces or patios of mosquitoes, make a mini-bonfire in a fireproof container – like an old tin; stuff it with grass or paper, and liberally sprinkle with some of the following dried herbs: Rue, Sage, Southernwood, Wormwood, Rosemary, Cedar, Elecampane.

MOTHS

Of all the essential oils, Camphor is perhaps the least attractive to the human nose. I remember coming across the little frosty-white balls of Camphor among my mother's clothes, and wondering why she chose to have anything that smelled so nasty near them. Everybody now associates the smell of Camphor with mangy furs, black cloth coats that have gone green with age, and cashmere sweaters worn to a cobweb.

Fortunately, there are alternatives. Dr Valnet suggests oil of Clove, Lavender, or Lemon; if you impregnate sachets of Lavender with a few drops of any of these oils, you will get double protection.

An early English suggestion, in Banckes' *Herbal*, was for Rosemary, 'Take the flowers and put them in a chest among your clothes or among books, the moth shall not hurt them.'

Danièle Ryman has an even more attractive idea: oil of Vetiver, a perfume in itself. In Russia, she says, wealthy women used to have tiny sachets of oil of Vetiver sewn into the linings of their expensive fur coats. She suggests putting sheets of blotting paper sprinkled with the oil in drawers and wardrobes.

In her lovely book *Pot-Pourris and Other Fragrant Delights*, Jacqueline Heriteau gives an adaptation of an old French recipe for a Sweet Bag to repel moths: 1 cup each of dried Rosemary, Tansy, Thyme, Mint, 1 cup Southernwood, ½cup ground Cloves. Chop and mince all the herbs together, and mix with the Cloves. Pour into little muslin bags.

Euell Gibbons has the most attractive idea of all. For the protection of his big, patterned Scandinavian wool sweaters, he lines a drawer with paper, sprinkles a mix of 1 pound of Pine needles, 25g/1oz of Cedar shavings, and about 12g/½oz Sassafras root shavings. He covers them with a layer of cloth – an old sheet, perhaps – thumbtacked into place. 'Your woollens . . . ,' he says, 'will not only be protected from depredations of moths, but will come out with a clean, masculine fragrance that fairly shouts of forests, mountains and the great manly outdoors.'

THE SWEET-SMELLING HOME

One of the first things you notice about a house is its smell. Stuffy and dusty, with stale cookery smells hanging around the hall? Sterile-clean, with a hospital reek of disinfectant or bleach? 'Fragranced' out of an aerosol? Warm and welcoming, with a hint of candles, flowers, logs on the fire?

There is plenty you can do to make your home an agreeable place to be, for yourself and your friends alike.

Choose cleaning materials that do *not* come perfumed with synthetic Roses, Lemon or Lavender; the 'Green' ranges often have very little smell, other than cleanness – another reason for choosing them.

When entertaining friends – especially if there are smokers among them – be lavish with candles. Candles seem to 'digest' any lingering odours, and keep the room smelling fresh and clean; in Amsterdam, there is always a candle burning in their famous Brown Bars. In Britain, we neglect the potential of candles – Scandinavian countries burn 20 candles to our 1. Candles used to be made from the waxy coating of the Wax Myrtle berry – sometimes known as the Candleberry – or the Bay berry,

gathered and made just before Christmas, with which their wonderful smell became associated. Today, you can buy candles loose or in tins or beautiful glass containers, already perfumed with essential oils for environmental fragrance.

Even minute amounts of an essential oil can fill a room with a lingering hint of some good smell. To diffuse it round the room, you can put 2-3 drops on a vaporizing ring round a light-bulb (see Useful Addresses, p.158, for suppliers). Or use an essential oil burner, in which a nightlight keeps warm a small saucer of water to which you add 2-3 drops of your oil. Or you can add 2-3 drops to a plant-mister half-filled with warm water and spray it around the room. Otherwise simply put a small bowl of water near or on top of a radiator and add the oils to the water. Use your favourite oil, or try Cedarwood, a smoky, rather masculine smell; warm spicy Frankincense for a party; Mountain Pine, fresh and woody; cleansing green Juniper. (Juniper twigs and sprigs of Rosemary used to be burnt together in French hospitals for their antiseptic powers.)

I use a plant-mister to spray pillow-cases, sheets, lingerie and my favourite blouses when I iron them – and add a couple of drops of my favourite Geranium oil. Lavender could be a classic choice. Jasmine or Ylang-Ylang would be very exotic. If you have a spin-drier, you can put a drop of oil on a hanky and add it to the load before drying.

To give your sitting-room the sweet elusive fragrance of a flower-garden, consider a pot-pourri.

POT-POURRI

Pot-pourri is newly fashionable. It is sold everywhere, but most of it looks as frightful as it smells; shavings of wood, fake buds and leaves dyed lurid pinks, yellows and greens give out a rank and insistent odour.

Even true pot-pourri, properly made, soon loses its elusive scent, since it is usually displayed in beautiful, wide dishes standing around the room. Left out in the open like this, pot-pourri soon fades, gathers dust and loses its fragrance.

Traditionally, pot-pourri should be kept in big, closed jars, with a well-fitting lid, under which is a perforated china lid. Just before the room is to be used, the jar is opened, and warmed at the fire or in the sun, to release its subtle aromas into the room. Kept closed like this, a good pot-pourri will last for years.

There is a lot of mystique surrounding the making of pot-pourri; if you live in a tiny flat without even a balcony to fill with plant-pots, it is probably better to buy good ready-made pot-pourri from one of the growing number of good suppliers (see Useful Addresses, p.158). The same suppliers, however, also sell the individual ingredients – including all the dried flower petals, leaves, spices, and fixatives – so you could still have a go.

If you live in the country and have your

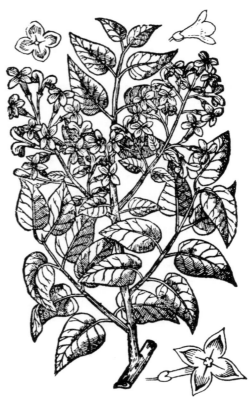

own garden it is worth trying your hand at a simple pot-pourri just to get the feel of it. (Like making your own bread or mayonnaise, making pot-pourri sounds more complicated than it actually is.)

Forget about the complex, moist pot-pourris, the ones Elizabethan ladies of the manor produced, in which semi-dried petals and leaves ferment in a mix of salt to produce entirely different scents.

Dry pot-pourri is made with leaves and flower-petals collected over weeks and months and dried till they crackle. Then they are mixed together, a fixative and a fragrant oil added. The mixture is left to rest, infuse and develop its own characteristic flavour.

Among the flowers and plants that look and smell nice in a pot-pourri are the following: Roses (essential – and some of them should be in bud form); Syringa; Jasmine; Clove Pinks; Stock; Phlox; Lavender; Rosemary; Mint;

Sage; Thyme; Marjoram; Lemon Verbena. Petals from cut flowers or pot plants can be added too.

Bay leaves, Pine cones and dried Orange peel will help give a spicier mix; most of the kitchen spices are traditional additions to revive a fading perfume.

The petals should be absolutely dry when picked, or they could rot and spoil your entire collection. Petals and leaves need to be dried as you go along, spread out on sheets of newspaper in an airy room. Judy Almond, who supplies pot-pourri to the National Trust and a number of stately homes, collects hers into a garden sieve lined with muslin; she keeps the sieve handy near the boiler, dropping petals and leaves into it as they come to hand. When they are crackly dry, she moves them into a big cardboard box near the boiler until it is time to make up her pot-pourri, giving them a stir from time to time.

When you have collected and dried enough for your pot-pourri, you will need a fixative, which helps 'fix' the various perfumes of the mixture, a number of spices to give their warm base notes; and a fragrant oil to pull all the perfumes together and give them body.

The classic fixatives – Storax, Gum Benzoin, Orris root, Sweet Flag or Violet Root Powder – need to be ordered from a herbal supplier, and sound pricey. A little goes a long way, though; a couple of teaspoons of Orris root, for instance, will 'fix' the contents of a big bowl of dried material.

Instead of these exotic fixatives, you can use citrus peel. Judy Almond collects Orange, Lemon and Tangerine peel and puts it near the boiler to dry, then grinds it to powder in a coffee mill.

There are no set rules for the composition of a pot-pourri: you choose the ingredients and the combination of scents that most appeal.

For the spices, choose from: Cloves, Star Anise (very popular because they look so attractive); Cinnamon sticks; Juniper berries; Bay leaves; whole Nutmegs; and Cardamom.

The oil should be one of the more fragrantly appealing: Geranium; Rose; Neroli; Lemon; Ylang-Ylang; or Lavender. For a more intriguing spicy smell, try: Vetiver; Cypress; Cedar; Melissa; or Nutmeg. Use a tiny amount of this oil – no more than 8–10 drops at most for every big bowl of pot-pourri. Add this to the fixative before stirring them both into the mix.

Once you have got your dried plant material, bought or made the fixative, and chosen the oil, you are ready to *make* your pot-pourri.

'I use a large old plastic washing-up bowl to mix the pot-pourri,' Judy Almond explains in *The Herbalist*, 'and I keep a small bowl and old spoon especially to mix the oils and powdered peel together, otherwise my family complain that even the gravy tastes scented.'

Dried material, oil, fixative and the spices of your choice should be thoroughly sifted together. Add the spices a little at a time, sniffing as you go along; no one smell should overwhelm the mixture.

When you are happy with your pot-pourri, transfer to a sealable wooden or cardboard box and leave in a warm place for 4–6 weeks to mature. Sniff occasionally to see how it is doing.

Pot-pourris can have a single scent or colour theme. Mrs Imogen Nichols, who sells hers at Open Gardens to raise money for the church, and supplies it to the local Museum shop, makes a Lavender one, a Lemon one, a golden one and a silver one, depending on what happens to be growing well in her herb garden at the time. 'All my pot-pourris are herbal,' she says, 'I feel that everyone makes the Rose petal one.'

When she collects the herbs she dries them

hanging up in bunches on the landing – 'nice and airy'. Once dried, they are stored in re-cycled supermarket brown-paper bags till she is ready to rub them. Then they are mixed with a little Orris root, and stored in glass jars in the dark until she is ready to make the pot-pourri.

For the Lemon one use anything lemony. Lemon Balm; Lemon Verbena; Lemon Thyme and Mint; Geraniums; a twist of dried Lemon peel; Lemon-scented Hypericum; Pennyroyal;

or a little Mint, but not very much. Try Bay leaves scrunched up, and a few Santolina flowers to decorate. 'I put a piece of Lemon Grass in the sweet jars where I store the dried herbs,' Mrs Nichols says.

The silver one – a useful fly-repellant – is made from the silvery-coloured *Artemisias*; Wormwood and Southernwood; variegated Apple Mints (for grey colour); Lemon Balm; Grey Sage, but not too much; Bay leaves, crunched; and Eidelweiss to decorate.

DISINFECTANTS

In the kitchen, the bathroom and the sick-room, herbs can protect us against infective micro-organisms. Especially effective are the marvellous aromatic plants – Rosemary, Ori-gan, Thyme, Sage and others – which have been used by housewives for centuries to pre-vent food putrefying, as well as to ward off in-fection. When these antiseptic powers were first seriously studied in the laboratory, from the late nineteenth century onwards, the find-ings were remarkable. As just one example: an aqueous solution of the essential oil of Thyme kills the typhus bacillus, and Shiga's bacillus – responsible for epidemic dysentery – in 2 minutes; streptococcus and the diptheria bacil-lus within 4, and the tuberculosis bacillus in 30-60 minutes.

In some thought-provoking French experi-ments, a blend of aromatic essences – Pine, Thyme, Peppermint, Lavender, Rosemary, Cloves and Cinnamon – was tested for the bac-teriological purification of a closed environ-ment, containing numbers of moulds, staphy-lococci and assorted micro-organisms in open Petri dishes. Within 30 minutes of being sprayed with the aromatic mix, all the moulds and staphylococci had been wiped out; of the

original 210 microbial colonies, a mere 4 re-mained. The potential for use in hospitals – where cross-infections are a growing and deadly threat – is huge. Let us hope that it may some day be exploited.

Meanwhile, we can at least protect ourselves from domestic infections. When cleaning out your fridge, freshen it with a quick wipe-round of water into which you have squeezed the juice of a Lemon.

Make a strong infusion of Thyme or Rose-mary – a handful of the herb infused covered in a good mugful of boiling water – and use it to wipe down the shelves of the store-cupboard or larder when next you have a clean-out.

Bathroom and cloakroom floors can be mopped with water to which you add a couple of drops of Tea Tree oil.

If somebody in the family is in bed with an infectious illness – the first winter case of 'flu, perhaps – exploit the anti-viral and anti-bacte-rial properties of the great aromatic herbs. Put 2 or 3 drops of the essential oils of Clary Sage, Geranium and Lavender, in a plant-mister half-filled with water, and spray it around the the sickness. (**N.B.** I keep the plant-mister just for essential-oil use of this kind).

IN THE KITCHEN

At the beginning of the ninth century, the newly-proclaimed Emperor Charlemagne promulgated a Decree (Capitulare de Villis): the Decree Concerning Principal Cities. It laid down that in every important city of the Empire, gardens should be laid out planted with 'all herbs' as well as certain trees and fruits.

The 73 'herbs' listd included a number described as 'Physical' – grown chiefly for medicinal purposes. Among them are many which today would be thought of only as culinary, such as Sage, Rosemary and Fennel. This was a purely administrative distinction, however; it was intended for those in charge of large estates or monasteries, where a separate Physic Garden would be kept, as well as kitchen and pleasure gardens.

VERT SAUSE

Take parsel, and myntes, and peletur, and costmaryn, and sauge, and a lytel garlek and bredde, and grinde hit smal, and tempur hit up with vynegur, and do therto pouder of pepur, and of Gynger, and of canel, and serve hit forthe.

A Roll of Ancient Cookery AD 1331
(Ed. The Revd. Richard Warner,
Antiquitates Culnariae).

For the housewife, the distinction between a herb cultivated for the kitchen and table, and a herb grown for medicinal purposes, was non-existent. Rosemary might be prescribed 'for weyknesse of ye brayne' or because it was 'a remedy for the windiness in the stomach, bowels and spleene, and expels it powerfully'. But what country housewife could do without Rosemary to make her lard or roast lamb tasty, or flavour her ales and wines?

Sage might well be 'useful in the deflucions of rheum in the head, and for diseases of the chest or breast'; it was just as indispensable in the kitchen to make Sage and Onion stuffing for a goose, or flavour a special cheese.

Home remedies were sometimes administered in the form of a wry-tasting potion. Just as often, though, they were dished up in the more agreeable shape of food or drink – caudles and possets, gruels and green pottages, sacks, ales, beers and wines brewed from herbs.

There was an awareness that specific foods could be healing in specific ways. The *Regimen Sanitatis*, a long rhyming treatise on health and diet which was widely read throughout Europe during the later Middle Ages, spelled out item by item the virtues or otherwise of various fruits, vegetables and herbs. The Nettle 'helps him of the Goute that eates it often . . . . Of Fennel, The stomach it doth cleanse and comfort welle'.

Some of these beliefs were expressions of medical prejudice; in the fifth century the influential physician Galen denounced raw fruit as an unhealthy article of diet; the prejudice lingered in medical circles, and in wealthy eating habits, for nearly a millennium.

More often, belief in the medicinal powers of certain foods was based on centuries of experience and hearty country cooking traditions, at a level of society that had no money to spend on grand physicians.

These healing powers were exploited – often almost unconsciously – in the meals planned for any household: in the springtime 'green drinks' made with vitamin-C rich herbs that banished winter-time scurvy; in the fermented foods and the herbal ales that aided digestion; in the aromatic Garlic and Sage broths that helped ward off chest infections.

Eating in season by necessity not choice, people ate more healthily too. The changing seasons each bring foodstuffs appropriate to the time of year. The cooling fruits and salads, the flowers and green herbs of summer give way to the sustaining grains, berries, and nuts of autumn. More substantial still are the starchy root vegetables of winter; the dried fruits often made up into soothing Pectoral drinks; the sulphur-rich Onions, Cabbages and Leeks that help keep respiratory systems clear in the season of frost and snow; and the warming spices added to puddings and drinks. And so to

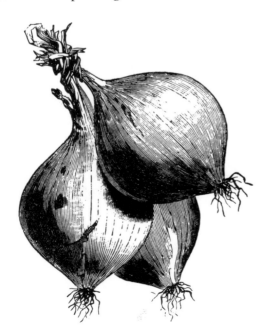

spring, with its bursting greens and tender young vegetables.

With no exotic fruits or overseas markets to draw on, local resources and the rich diversity of nature were fully exploited, adding variety to meals, furnishing medicines or serving domestic purposes. Every household was Green by necessity – economy and ecology went hand in hand. Many of the plants used served several different purposes.

Flowers were used as decoration or colouring for food; blossoms turned up in wines and fritters, buds were boiled in puddings or pickled as a relish. Healing herbs were brewed up into beers and wines, the roots and stems of medicinal plants were candied to produce sweetmeats; the leaves and barks might furnish dyes as well as drugs. The tea-time conserve might be added to hot water to make a cough cure; the ale was often a cure for scurvy or constipation; the flower-based vinegar used for a salad also served as a gargle for a sore throat or a tonic for the complexion.

Any idea that the limitations of eating locally and in season-imposed monotony on the diet of centuries before the refrigerator and the deep freeze cannot survive a look at the evidence. Witness the Receipt books of the sixteenth and seventeenth centuries. On the contrary, the range and variety of foods and flavours is striking.

In Madam Bridget Hyde's Receipt book, kept over 14 years from 1676 onwards, the recipes written in her fine flowing hand include: Birch, Gooseberry or Apricock Wine; Sirrup of Mulberries; Wild Carrot Ale; Candied Barberries; Thyme Cream, Sirrops of Violettes and many others.

Charlemagne's Decree listed 5 different categories of Apple: Sweetings, Sour Apples, Keepers, Earlies, and those for instant eating – each with a number of different Apples in it. In the seventeenth century Parkinson could name over 50 different varieties. Medlars, Quinces and Apricocks were all being grown in England in the eighteenth century. In no month were there fewer than half-a-dozen varieties of Apple available, and Pears were almost as numerous.

When Thomas Tusser listed the Herbs that might be grown on a Tudor estate in the mid-sixteenth century, he named 43 'Seedes and Herbes for the Kitchen' including several we should class as vegetables, and others we should never think of cooking with today, such as Avens, Burnet and Tansy. He listed a further 22 'Herbes and Rootes for Sallets and Sauce' of which a few are just creeping back into use – Purslane, or 'Rokat' – and others which you hardly ever hear of – Alexanders, Ramsons, or Skirret.

In *Lark Rise to Candleford*, Flora Thompson described a small agricultural community in the 1880s, where everyone was so poor that meat seldom appeared on their tables. Yet they feasted on the vegetables the men grew on their allotments – 'there was always competition amongst them as to who should have the earliest and choicest of each kind. . . . ' They were fussy about their potatoes, growing 'all the old-fashioned varieties – ashleaf kidney, early rose, American rose, magnum bonum and the huge misshaped white elephant'.

Freshness and variety are the stuff of gourmet eating, and are also vital to our health. Foods are not simply attractively-presented packages of well-known nutrients – they are wonderful complexes of a myriad natural chemicals. Scientists today, putting one common foodstuff after another under the microscope, are uncovering a staggering range of therapeutic substances. Their findings often confirm the instinctive wisdom of country eating traditions. But they do little more than hint

at the healing wealth around us, in fruits, vegetables, grains, nuts and seeds, in herbs and spices, and in the Wild Foods we leave to rot on the trees or in the hedgerows.

The pages that follow are an introduction and a tribute to that wealth and variety.

WHAT IS HEALTHY EATING?

Healthy food is enjoyable food, good enough to be eaten and savoured slowly. It should offer a spectrum of tastes to please our palates: sweet, sour, salty, spicy, pungent, bitter.

It is food which reaches our tables as soon as possible after harvesting, wherever possible grown without agrochemicals.

Food should be eaten in its whole, natural form, such as brown Rice, whole Wheat, unrefined vegetable oils, fruits and vegetables with the skins on.

Finally, healthy food is free of the chemical additives which can give it unnatural colour, flavour, texture or shelf-life.

This is food at its best; it is not always available, and often costs more than you can afford, unless you grow your own. This is still the quality you should aim at, however.

Try delicious, nutty wholewheat bread, and you might even start making your own. Brown Rice, Oats, Millet – too good to leave strictly for the birds – and Pot Barley should all find their way to your table.

At least once a day, eat a big helping of green vegetables, with their high content of health-giving chlorophyll, vitamins and minerals. Eat brightly coloured vegetables such as Tomatoes, Carrots, Pumpkin, Beetroot, Peppers, Red Cabbage, Radishes too for the vital antioxidant, beta-carotene. Salad made from fresh raw vegetables and sprouted seeds is a must, as is plenty of fresh fruit, if possible eaten in season.

For variety try including Wild Food in your

menu – Hips and Haws, Rowanberries, Elderberries, Blackberries, Dandelion, and Chickweed, for example.

Enjoy pure extra-virgin Olive oil – one of the most wonderfully healthy foodstuffs of the Mediterranean – or if possible cold-pressed, unrefined Sunflower oil and some butter for your fat needs. From time to time eat a piece of one of our splendid native cheeses.

You need good quality protein: beef, lamb and free-range poultry; eat fresh eggs too, if possible from free-range hens.

If you are vegetarian, plan your meals carefully to make up the protein and essential nutrients not supplied by meat or fish.

Include in your dishes fresh whole Nuts in their autumn and winter season, and Sunflower and Sesame seeds, all rich sources of protein and mineral.

You can add zest and seasoning to your eating with nature's vast range of wonderful herbs and spices.

With your evening meal you might enjoy a glass of good wine. Or as an *aperitif* or *digestif* there is nothing better than a medicinal wine you have prepared yourself.

This is Slow Food, for quality eating. The following section of this book will tell you much more about what wonderful foods like these can do for you and your health, offering suggestions on how to prepare and enjoy them.

. . . it will be found, whatever additions may be made to our knowledge, that all elements and complexes necessary for normal nutrition – so far as food can provide them – are present in the fresh fruits of the Earth as Nature furnishes them; though not in these foodstuffs as man mishandles and maltreats them.
from 'Introductory Remarks on Nutrition Today', Nutrition, 1947

(Sir Robert McCarrison)

HERBS

'The friend of physicians and the pride of cooks' – this description of herbs has been attributed to the Emperor Charlamagne, a noted enthusiast.

Throughout the centuries, the herbs we tend to think of today as purely culinary have often served this dual purpose. To this end, they were lavishly added to soups, stews, salads, omelettes and other made-up dishes – with what we might consider a fairly heavy hand.

In the Middle Ages omelettes made with chopped herbs were popular. Unlike our modern *omelette fines herbes*, though, the *herbolace*, as it was called by French cooks, was almost as solid as a Spanish *tortilla*, so great was the quantity of herbs added. The Goodman of Paris gave his wife careful instructions on how to make one, and which herbs to use, in a nicely calculated gradation of flavours.

The thick green mixture was fried in oil and butter well heated in a frying pan, and turned to cook on both sides; grated cheese was added on top. When this had melted the *herbolace* was allowed to cool a little, then dished up.

Both Dittany and Tansy are herbs with a powerful, pungent taste; and modern taste would probably leave out the Ginger.
Richard II's cookery book, the *Forme of Cury* was written around the same time as the

Goodman of Paris' treatise. One of its recipes is for a baked omelette called an *Erbolate*; similar to the Paris version, it uses many of the same herbs. The herbs are finely chopped, mixed with eggs, put in a buttered dish and baked.

Take of Dittany two leaves only, and of Rue less than half or naught, for know that it is strong and bitter; of Smallage, Tansy, Mint and Sage, of each four leaves or less, for each is strong; Marjoram a little more, Fennel more, Parsley more still, but of Porray, Beets, Violet leaves, Spinach, Lettuces and Clary, as much of the one as of the others, until you have two large handfuls. Pick them over and wash them in cold water, then dry them of all the water and bray two heads of Ginger. And then have sixteen eggs well beaten together, yolks and whites, and bray them and mix them in the mortar with the things aforesaid, then divide it into two, and make two thick omelettes.

The Goodman of Paris
(Eileen Power (ed))

For centuries the basic food of the European peasantry was a thick, starchy soup, based on Oatmeal, Barley, dried Peas or Beans. Chopped green vegetables and herbs gave it variety and flavour. For the better off, the liquid might be a chicken, mutton or veal broth, with a beaten-up yolk of egg sometimes added to thicken it.

These pottages were often intentionally medicinal: in *The Leechbook of Bald* – a tenth century Anglo-Saxon medical treatise – 'juicy broths' were often a carefully prescribed part of the treatment: Garlic for constipation, Radishes and Elecampane with Barley for lung complaints among them.

In Medieval times, the pottage – or *porray*, because it was usually based on Leeks – might have had any number of seasonal herbs and vegetables added to it – a useful source of minerals and vitamins – as well as the protective qualities supplied by the herbs. Parsley was a prime favourite; every cottager took care to have a little patch of it. Even the poorest little gardens were usually well-stocked with herbs, and the countryside could supply dozens more. Among favourite Medieval pot-herbs, supplying a range of flavours mild, bitter, savoury, hot or sharp, were: Savory; Fennel; Dandelion; Nettles; Sage; Thyme; Chives; Marigolds; two pungent, aromatic plants – Alexanders and Lovage; Avens – an aromatic and tonic herb; and Smallage – a kind of wild celery. Beet, Mallows and Orache supplied large green leaves to give substance to the *porray*.

As late as the seventeenth century, herb and vegetable pottages were part of every good housewife's repertoire; for the tables of the rich, though, meat was always the basis of the broth, and the starchy thickening was supplied by slices of bread at the bottom of the pot. The herbs used were fresh, not dried, and in season. The cooling summer herbs would produce a lighter, sharp-tasting broth; in medicine, the same herbs would be prescribed to counter fevers, indigestion and liver problems. The warming aromatic herbs of the winter pottage would help counter colds, chilliness, lung problems and rheumatism.

The greens served up for an English country dinner often took the form of a herb pudding, which might be made with a variety of herbs or vegetables: Cabbage; Cauliflower; Kale; Broccoli; Watercress; Onions; Dandelions or Dock leaves were used. Wild herbs with a sharp or bitter taste, such as Bistort or Lady's Mantle, combined with Oatmeal, Barley or both were also popular. They were boiled in a pudding-basin tied with a cloth, to make a substantial accompaniment to meat, or to be enjoyed on their own.

The young shoots of Bistort, with their sharp flavour, were particularly popular in Cumberland or Westmoreland, where this plant grows freely in moist meadowland. They were combined with young Nettle tops to make a healthy spring-time dish.

HERB POTTAGE

Take Elder buds, nettle tops, clivers and watercress, and what quantity of water you please proportionable to your quantity of herbs, add oatmeal according as you would have it in thickness and when your water and oatmeal is just ready to boyl, put your herbs into it, cut or uncut as you like best; take a Ladle and ladle it and then you may eat it with the herbs or strain it adding a little butter, salt and bread. The best will be not to eat it till it is somewhat cooled and not past as hot as milk from the cow. You are to remember not to let it boyl at all. This is a brave, wholesom cleansing sort of pottage far beyond what is commonly made.

The Good Housewife
(T. Tryon, 1692)

NB. This healthy soup features 4 herbs any housewife could have gathered in the countryside in the spring: cleansing and nutrient-rich. The herbs are added only briefly to the not-quite-boiling soup, so much of their vitamin C will survive, too.

BISTORT PUDDING

Allow about 1½lb of Bistort to 1lb of Nettles. A few leaves of Black Currant and Yellow Dock may be added and a sprig of Parsley. Wash the vegetables thoroughly (in salt and water in the last rinsing) then chop them fairly fine. Place them in a bowl and mix in about a teacupful of Barley (washed and soaked), half a teacupful of Oatmeal, salt and pepper to flavour, and if liked, a bunch of chives mixed. Boil the whole in a bag for about 2½ hours, to allow the Barley to get thoroughly cooked. The bag should be tied firmly, for while the greens shrink, the barley swells. Turn out into a very hot bowl, add a lump of butter and a beaten egg: the heat of the turned-out pudding is sufficient to cook the egg.

A Modern Herbal
(Mrs M. Grieve, 1931)

Green salads were eaten enthusiastically in England from Roman times; the range and variety of herbs used – either as seasoning or to make up the salad – was staggering. A salad served at Richard II's table in the late fourteenth century was made of: Parsley, Sage, Garlic, Chives, Onions, Leeks, Borage, Mints, Fennel and Cresses, dressed with oil and vinegar. In Elizabethan times salads became more elaborate, garnished with hard-boiled eggs and slices of Cucumber and with the flowers Borage, Primrose or Violet which gave colour to Medieval salads.

In the late seventeenth century John Evelyn listed no less than 82 herbs and greens that might feature in a salad. Some of them, such as Purslane and Rocket, are just coming back into culinary fashion today, others are unfamiliar even by name – Jack by the Hedge, Orach, Skirrets and Sowthistle.

The Victorian age saw the steady decline of the Englishman's food, and the skilful use of herbs declined with it. The recipes in Victorian and Edwardian cookery books often look curiously bare; herbs are conspicuous by their absence; bland was becoming a national favourite, occasionally contrasted with sharp, vinegary sauces.

Fortunately, the last few decades are seeing a deepening British interest in food and cookery. An enormous range of dried herbs and spices is now available in every supermarket, many of them selling a good variety of fresh herbs, too. Most garden centres also sell a wide range of herbs. If you have neither enterprizing supermarket nor well-stocked garden centre within reach, you can order plants by post, some of them organically grown. It is worth growing your own, even if you only have space for a few favourites in pots on a sunny window-sill.

The essential oils of aromatic herbs like Thyme, Rosemary and Tarragon can be potent medicines but the use of the plants themselves can be the best kind of preventive medicine for our digestions, respiratory systems, our hearts, or stressed nerves. Recent research has demonstrated the existence of antioxidants in the essential oils of these culinary herbs, too, which makes them particularly useful in our polluted age and almost all of them have some level of anti-infective activity, giving us year-round protection against infectious disease, and preserving us from the food poisoning which is becoming epidemic today.

BASIL

This herb came to Europe from India, where it is a revered plant, sacred to both Krishna and Vishnu. In the Mediterranean, Basil soon went native – it is hard to imagine the *cuisine* of Provence or northern Italy without this piercingly aromatic plant. On the south-facing Ligurian hills near Genoa grows – it is claimed – the best and sweetest Basil in Italy; *pesto*, that wonderful pasta sauce made of pounded Basil, Garlic, Pine-nuts, pecorino cheese and Olive oil, is a local speciality. Provence is equally proud of its *Soupe au Pistou* – a Bean and vegetable soup enriched at table with spoonfuls of Pistou – Garlic and Basil again. Basil and Tomatoes, the deep red ones that have ripened naturally in strong sunshine, is another of the great gastronomic partnerships; add mozzarella cheese and a dribble of Olive oil for a tri-coloured salad that says summer to my eyes.

Basil prospers in plenty of sunshine; appropriately, this sunshine plant has for centuries been considered a tonic for melancholy and low spirits. Its anti-spasmodic qualities make it useful in headaches, the insomnia that comes from stress and tension, and nervous indigestion. If you want to indulge yourself, take Basil in the form of an alcoholic extraction: add a handful of leaves to a litre of good red wine, leave to macerate for 3 days, strain and sip a small glassful after dinner.

BAY

Bay was for heroes in ancient times, who were crowned with a wreath of its leaves. In both cooking and medicine, a little Bay goes a long way. A single leaf will lend its distinctive aroma to a whole panful of soup, or perfume a savoury bean stew. A Bay leaf is one of the ingredients of the classic *bouquet garni*. As it is powerfully antiseptic, I tuck a Bay leaf or two inside a chicken or under a piece of meat before storing it in the refrigerator.

Bay leaves are a tonic for the whole system. After an attack of fever, or chronic bronchitis, make this cold-weather infusion. Pour a cupful of water over a small Bay leaf and a couple of pieces of dried Orange peel; cover and leave to infuse for 15 minutes. Sweeten with a little honey and sip.

Bay grows freely all round the Mediterranean, and if you holiday there, you may well be able to harvest and carry home a whole year's supply. Be very careful that it is true Bay, however; the leaves of the look-alike Cherry Laurel can be poisonous.

CHERVIL

This is one of the most interesting and delicious of the kitchen herbs, with a flavour not unlike Parsley. Bruise a leaf between your fingers and you will sniff that delicate whiff of Aniseed, too.

This is a herb to be used liberally: in salads, stews, omelettes, buttery sauces, and in simple Potato soups enriched with cream. Together with Beet tops, Sorrel and Lettuce it used to feature in a green *bouillon*, a cleansing and refreshing remedy for persistent constipation. The juice of Chervil was mixed with wild Chicory, Lettuce and Dandelion for a liver tonic. It is a cleansing herb, and a cheering tonic.

It should be used fresh and green, never dried.

Chervil water was once distilled by every housewife, as a valued cosmetic aid; it helped clear the skin of blemishes, soothing reddened and inflamed eyes. French doctors today suggest it as an eyewash for ophthalmic problems, and in the treatment of wrinkles or greasy skin.

CHIVES

Chives are the mild, well-bred member of the common Onion family. They share all the health-giving properties of the family – antiseptic, good for the digestion of rich foods, a protection for the respiratory system. If you are sensitive – as many people claim to be – to Onions or Garlic, you should still be able to enjoy Chives without discomfort. Eat plenty of them, chopped into fresh, green, summer salads, added to a simple *omelette fines herbes*; sprinkled into cold soups such as Vichyssoise, and as a wonderful garnish – with plenty of Parsley – for a Tomato salad. They also taste delicious added to home-made Mayonnaise, and are a good alternative to spring onions.

DILL

The feathery fronds of Dill turn up in fish cookery all over Scandinavia, and in cream cheeses, soups, and Potato salads. Its little seeds are warming and comforting to the windy stomach; an infusion of them – a teaspoonful in a cup of boiling water, infused for 6 minutes covered – is a folk remedy for hiccups.

The name derives from a Scandinavian word meaning 'to lull', which is what it does to a digestive system in turmoil. It may well have been the first herbal remedy you ever tried, in the form of Gripe Water, given to windy babies.

GARLIC

Imagine a new wonder-drug which could help cure cases of pneumonia, bronchitis and tuberculosis; improve resistance to infectious disease; treat high blood pressure; lower cholesterol levels; act as a tonic to the heart and digestive system; diminish the chances of getting cancer; clear up urinary infections and infestation by worms; deal with ear infections; stop wounds turning septic; and keep old age at bay. All this is achieved with virtually zero toxicity. Any pharmaceutical company that announced the launch of such a drug would be greeted with howls of derision. I buy it in quantity at my greengrocer: Garlic, of course.

Just about every one of the healing actions described has been verified round the world in clinical studies of Garlic and its potent volatile oils.

Garlic preserved the lives and health of the slaves who toiled to build the Pyramids. While patrician Romans would have nothing to do with the offensive bulb, it was Garlic that kept the Roman Legions going; it sprang up wherever the Imperial armies established a garrison.

Garlic's one side-effect, bad breath, has lost it many friends, however. Even in countries where its awesome healing powers were admitted, it was often ignored by the ruling classes and the aristocracy, 'The duke would mouth with a beggar, though she smelt brown bread and garlic', says a courtier scornfully in *Measure for Measure*, summing up the Elizabethan attitude. A century later John Evelyn said, ' . . . we absolutely forbid it entrance into our Salleting, by reason of its intolerable rankness. . . . '

Whatever its medicinal properties, lovers of good food enjoy the rich gutsy topnote Garlic contributes to the sunsoaked cuisine of the Mediterranean; I cannot imagine eating without it.

HORSERADISH

'I do not think we make enough use of horseradish,' wrote Constance Spry in an elegant wartime volume, *Come into the Garden, Cook*. She suggested that we should try it, ' . . . with most fried food: fish, cutlets, croquettes of meat or fish, or vegetable fritters, and especially so with smoked trout or eel,' in addition to its inevitable appearance with roast beef. It could accompany grilled ham, be used in sandwiches, added to a creamy bread-sauce, or stirred into lightly whipped cream together with a spot of Mustard, and Tarragon vinegar.

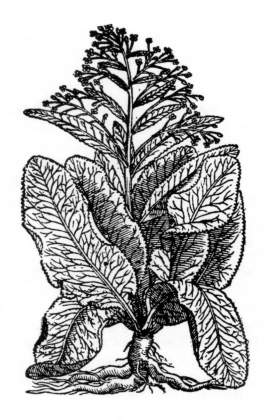

A little grated Horseradish can work wonders for a bland cottage-cheese salad, add piquancy to a dish of grated Carrots, or variety to a salad dressing. Try a dish of grated raw Beetroot, folded into a cream and Horseradish sauce with plenty of chopped Chives or Parsley. Always use the freshly grated root, not one of the made-up sauces sold in supermarkets.

Horseradish is powerful stuff, one of the sulphurous Crucifer family; too much of it can produce streaming eyes, headaches, and skin irritations. Some react to it with an upset stomach and if you are suffering from any kind of inflammatory disorder – piles, for instance, avoid it.

Rich in valuable minerals, including silica, it also contains enough vitamin C to make it a tried-and-tested cure for scurvy. Its healing powers in asthma, congested sinuses, catarrh, and lung infections can be dynamic. Try this for a sinus problem. Freshly-grated Horse-radish root is made into a thick pulp with a little cider vinegar, and a coffee-spoonful of it held in the mouth for as long as possible. Your eyes may water but your head will soon feel clear as a bell. For whooping cough, bronchi-tis, catarrh, take a regular spoonful dose before meals and at bedtime.

Horseradish is also recommended for both the elderly and the anaemic. As preventative medicine, and as a fine relish for our food, we should learn to appreciate this biting root.

Horseradish was another harbinger of spring, the first green thing to shove its rapier blades above the chilly earth. A few weeks later the lacquered emerald leaves would find their peppery way to the simple planning of our menus as 'greens', mixed with the milder-flavoured narrow dock which, with other edible weeds, grew outside the pale of their more civilised relations.

In the first pale days of early spring, however, its part was merely to lend zest as a relish to the diet. Washed, scraped, and grated – with salt, vinegar, and sugar added, and conserved in a glass jar – it was ready to be used on baked beans, salt pork, or corned beef.

The Country Kitchen
(Delia Lutes, 1938)

--- o ---

MARJORAM

Also known as Sweet Marjoram, it is closely related to Wild Marjoram, otherwise known as Origan, made famous worldwide in the omni-present pizza. Origan grows wild in Mediter-ranean countries; on hot sunny days in the hills, you may catch a wonderful whiff of its unique odour. In Andalucia, it is considered a cure-all by peasants; curiously enough, though, it does not feature in their cooking.

Beyond their wonderful aromas, and the sharp note they add to cookery, both are calm-ing, soothing herbs, and noted anti-spasmod-ics. Drink Marjoram tea when you are feeling edgy, nervy, irritable; when your stomach is filled with the butterflies of anxiety; or when tension is keeping you awake at night. Try it for spasmodic coughs, or menstrual cramps too. Marjoram features on singers' list of remedies to be tried when hoarseness threatens – they drink an infusion of Marjoram with honey. Marjoram wine – made by macerating 50g/2oz fresh herbs in a litre of good red wine for a fortnight, then filtered – can be an ex-cellent *digestif* or sleep-inducer. Enjoy a small glass of it after dinner.

MINTS

Think of English cookery, and you automati-cally think of roast lamb with mint sauce. In the cookery books attributed to the Roman gourmet Apicius, however, fresh or dried mint sauces crop up constantly. Mint is com-bined with Cumin seeds and roasted Pine-nuts in a sauce for roast pork; with Onion, Dates and Coriander for roast wood-pigeon; with Pepper, Origan, Almonds and Honey as a sauce for cold fish; and with Pepper, Lovage, red wine and vinegar to eat with 'wild sheep'.

The celebrated English Mint sauce is often vile and vinegary, artificially coloured bright green. Constance Spry suggests making it, in-stead, with equal quantities of a good vinegar and Orange juice, or adding melted Redcur-rant jelly to the finished sauce.

The marvellous Mint tea served to guests in Morocco after a delicious meal is made with green Tea and plenty of Spearmint.

Mint is full of vitamin C and all the goodness of greenery – beta-carotene and chlorophyll – so eat plenty of it chopped up very finely in salads. Huge amounts of Mint and Parsley are used in the Middle Eastern *tabbouleh*.

Spearmint, the common or garden kind, is the Mint most familiar to housewives. Connoisseurs often prefer Bowles' mint, with its woolly leaves and faint Apple fragrance, or the Pineapple and Eau-de-Cologne variety; for medicinal tisanes, choose the purple-stemmed Peppermint.

All Mints are astringent, and of warm subtle parts; great strengtheners of the stomach. Their fragrance betokens them cephalics; they effectually take off nauseousness and retchings to vomit; they are also of use in looseness . . . the simple water, given to children, effectually removes the gripes; but these virtues more particularly belong to Sper and Peppermint.

The Complete Herbal
(Nicholas Culpeper)

In the Ancient World, Mint was medicine as much as condiment, valued as a stimulating tonic to the mind and the appetite. In a fascinating experiment in the USA recently, whiffs of the essential oil of Peppermint were shown to improve alertness in test subjects carrying out repetitive computer tasks by up to 30 per cent.

Mint is the perfect anti-spasmodic. A cup of Peppermint tea – and you can buy it in teabag form in any supermarket now – will allay gripes, cramps and spasms, or soothe nausea. Herbalists recommend it for morning sickness in pregnancy. For travel sickness, take a little dropper-bottle of Peppermint oil with you on your journeys, and put 2 drops in half a glass of water. Or take a thermos of hot peppermint tea, to which you have added a little grated fresh Ginger root. Children with tummy-aches can often be soothed by a few sips of this magical tea.

N.B. Peppermint tea should not be drunk too often in pregnancy, although the occasional cup will do no harm.

At the first shiver of a cold, or a bout of 'flu, exploit another useful quality of mint: it is mildly diaphoretic, or perspiration-inducing. This accounts for the great cooling quality which makes Mint so popular in refreshing summer drinks, such as the famous Mint Julep of Kentucky; in the cool cucumber salad of Greece; or in the yogurt-based *raita* of India.

NASTURTIUM

These jolly red, yellow and orange flowers have recently been rediscovered by epicures as a piquant addition to a salad. Add the flowers or tender young leaves, or both. The fruits can be pickled and used as a change from Capers; add a handful of them to a jar of Cider vinegar, together with some Cloves, a few Peppercorns, a little Thyme or Origan, and a Bay leaf.

Nasturtiums are rich in sulphur, the great cleanser; their gaudy colours indicate the presence of the wonder-working carotenoid pigments. They also have powerful natural antibiotic activity. If you suffer from chronic catarrh, bronchitis or poor vision, enjoy them often in your salads.

PARSLEY

More Parsley gets thrown away than used; washing and chopping it finely is such a chore. This is a shame, since Parsley adds interest and a cheerful green note to the flavour of many dishes such as simple omelettes, salads, stuffings and burgers. It is the robust flavour in a *bouquet garni*, delicious scattered over a simple grilled steak or fish.

Food snobs claim that continental Parsley – thin, and spare-leaved – has a superior flavour. My preference is for the crispy, curly, dense-leaved kind sold in Britain; it is a glorious green – and far more quickly chopped.

Parsley is rich in iron as well as beta-carotene and chlorophyll. If you are run-down, fatigued, low in energy, anaemic or prone to infections, sprinkle plenty of chopped Parsley. It is an excellent diuretic too, helpful to those with kidney or bladder problems.

ROCKET

It is thanks to foodies – often maligned – that Rocket is once more appearing on Northern tables. Italian greengrocers sell two varieties – the thin, dark leaves of the wild, and the softer, more rounded leaves of the cultivated kind; both are stocked the year round. Either adds a sharp, delicious peppery flavour, as well as a warming quality, to a salad; you either love or leave it. Medieval monks had no choice in the matter: Rocket was considered dangerously aphrodisiac, and was banned from their gardens. Some French authorities still consider it a sexual stimulant as well as a good general tonic.

In a Roman restaurant I was once served papery thin slices of sweet mountain ham garnished with plenty of Rocket, crumbs of sweet fresh Parmesan cheese, and a dribble of Olive oil.

ROSEMARY

Rosemary is a powerful – not to say pushy – flavouring; and a mouthful of the spiky little leaves is disagreeable. Properly used, though, there is nothing like it. Rosemary with a roast of indigestible young spring lamb, Rosemary warmed in the Olive oil in which cubed Potatoes are to be baked golden, Rosemary for marinades, or to stuff poultry, or marinaded in oil or vinegar to lend its warm Southern aroma – these are just some of the ways to enjoy its wonderful, pungent flavour.

The first Rosemary plants reportedly arrived in this country, sent to Philippa, Queen of England, by her mother the Countess of Hainault, in the fourteenth century.

The emblem of fidelity and constancy, Rosemary was often worn by women in their bridal crowns for luck. It came also to signify remembrance, love faithful even beyond the grave; Ophelia's nosegay included it: 'There's Rosemary, that's for remembrance; Pray you, love, remember. . . .' For this reason, its beautiful bushes were often planted on the graves of loved ones.

The association of Rosemary with memory is not just poetic fancy. It is a cerebral tonic, a stimulant to the brain as well as the system generally. It is particularly valuable in those states of general debility which are accompanied by loss of memory, loss of smell, poor vision, strain and nervous tension. Modern research has shown that it enhances the cellular uptake of oxygen, which helps account for its favourable effect on the brain.

Medicinally, Rosemary deserves a book to itself. See Part 3, Remedies, for its use for respiratory and liver problems and for the digestion.

When you are tired, low and washed-out, add a strong infusion of Rosemary to a stimulating bath, and sip a cup of Rosemary tea while you enjoy it (see Tea-Time for how to make it.) If you are really run down, add 3-4 Rosemary sprigs to a bottle of good, old red wine, macerate for 15 days, strain and sip a small glassful before dinner.

SAGE

This herb is best-known to the English in the form of Sage and Onion stuffing for a goose or a rolled joint of pork. This is one more instance of the instinctive wisdom of long culinary tradition. Both Sage and Onions help in the digestion of rich fatty meat; lower cholesterol levels; are useful tonics to the liver; and both are antiseptic (if either meat were tainted, it could still be eaten with reasonable safety). Sage was used for centuries as one of a dozen different herb flavouring for ales; at the beginning of the nineteenth century, a Manchester man was recorded as offering his guests a choice of 9 different flavoured ales – Sage, Hyssop and Rosemary among them.

So great are the tonic and antiseptic powers of Sage that the Chinese used to trade 3 cases of their own China tea for 1 of Sage. The seventeenth century herbalist Sir John Hill stresses, however, that Sage should be gathered and used in the spring, when its flowers are just beginning to open, and, 'there is in their cups a fragrant resin . . . highly flavoured, balmy, delicate, and, to the taste, one of the most delicious cordials that can be thought, warm and aromatic.'

Sage, like Rosemary, can be overdone as a flavour; but in the fragrant Provençal broth *Aigo Bouido*, you notice only its wonderful strengthening aroma.

To make the soup bring a litre of water to the boil, add 6-8 fresh Sage leaves, and simmer for about 15 minutes. Then add half a dozen fat cloves of Garlic, Salt and Pepper, and a coffee-cupful of Olive oil; simmer for another 10 minutes. Have ready thick slices of rustic bread, baked or toasted, put them in soup plates, and pour the fragrant broth over them. Try adding the beaten up yolk of a couple of eggs, with 2 spoonfuls of the broth, just before

serving; do not let it boil again, though. You could use a chicken or vegetable stock instead of plain water. In mid-winter it will help keep you free of colds and 'flu. (See Tea-Time, p.52, for Sage tea.)

Take a little Sage, a little Balm, put it into a pan, slice a Lemon, peel and all, a few knobs of sugar, one glass of white wine; pour on these two or three quarts of boiling water; cover it and drink when thirsty. When you think it strong enough of the herbs take them out otherwise it will make it bitter.

The New Art of Cookery
(Richard Briggs, 1788)

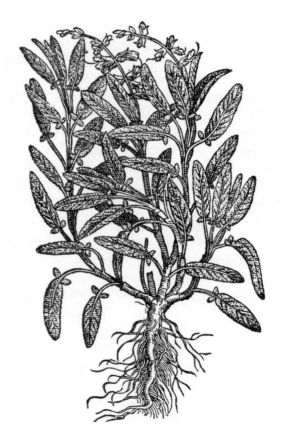

TARRAGON

This herb deserves to be used much more often than it is; most people only encounter it in the company of a roast chicken. Its fresh, aromatic taste can pep up sauces, mayonnaise, light soups – particularly a creamy Potato soup – and omelettes; and as Evelyn urged, 'the tops and young shoots like those of Rocket must never be excluded from sallets'.

A friendly herb, Tarragon calms digestive cramps and spasms; chew a leaf if you get the hiccups.

Make your own Tarragon vinegar as follows. Add a handful of leaves to a wide-mouthed jar; fill it with equal parts of white wine and a good vinegar, and let it macerate for 7-10 days. Then filter and rebottle.

THYME

Thyme is one of the quartet of savoury herbs which have survived in English cookery. Thyme and Parsley stuffing is a wonderfully robust accompaniment to roast chicken or turkey, and Thyme also flavoured the farmer's rabbit braised in cider. It went into some of the great game dishes, including partridge pudding, where the small joints together with slices of rump steak are steamed in a rich Thyme-flavoured stock. Thyme can be made into a savoury Apple jelly to serve with roast pork or chicken, and the agreeably fresh Lemon Thyme goes nicely with fish.

In the language of flowers, Thyme signifies courage, appropriate for a herb that can help you pick yourself up and get going again when you are low and run–down. Try this Italian tonic tea for instant uplift. Take a pinch of Thyme, a pinch of Angelica leaves or seeds, a pinch of Rosemary, and the peel of a well-scrubbed Orange; pour 2 cupfuls of boiling water over them, cover and let steep for 5 minutes. Then strain, and drink sweetened.

Country people often blended Thyme with Balm and Sage as a tea substitute – a very healthy brew. 'A noble strengthener of the lungs, as notable a one that grows,' wrote Culpeper enthusiastically, 'nor is there a better remedy for hooping cough'. Modern research has confirmed this judgment: for any convulsive cough, or lung problem, or today's mercifully rare cases of whooping cough, give plenty of Thyme tea. Take it, too, for all illnesses that start with a thorough chilling – sore throat, head colds, stiffness. Thyme is particularly valuable in 'flu – a powerful shot in the arm for the body's defence system.

PRESERVING HERBS

Many herbs can be dried successfully, and are easy to find in shops. However decorative those little pine spice-racks, the jars should be stored out of the light. Do not keep them too long; once they lose their distinctive aroma, you should throw them away.

Other herbs, however, only taste really good when fresh – Parsley, Basil, Chervil and Chives among them. You can freeze them for winter use. Strip them from their stalks and wash them carefully. Pat them lightly dry with kitchen paper, and seal into freezer bags from which you press out the air. Or you can add them in small quantities to an ice-cube tray; fill the tray with water, freeze it, and empty the cubes into a freezer bag. Label them carefully – one frozen green leaf looks very much like another.

Parsley and Chives can also be chopped very finely; store for freezing in lidded yogurt pots, from which you can scoop out a spoonful at a time for garnishing.

Herbal vinegars are another good way to store up the full summer flavour of fresh aromatic herbs, ready for instant use in soups, salads, or stews. Vinegar also extracts most of the medicinal properties of herbs. Specialty gourmet shops charge fortunes for those pretty little corked bottles housing a distinctive sprig of herb. You can make them much more cheaply at home – and give them away as presents too.

You need a wide-mouthed jar, preferably corked, or a kilner jar. The herb should be perfectly clean and dry. If absolutely necessary, wash it, but blot it bone-dry in plenty of kitchen paper. Then put it in the jar, which should be at least half-full, and fill the jar up with vinegar. Use a good Apple-cider vinegar for preference, or else a good white wine vinegar. Seal tightly, label, and store away in a dark place for at least a month. Then strain into a clean jug; coffee filter papers are the most efficient strainer. Put a fresh clean sprig of the herb into each of the jars you are going to fill, and pour in the strongly-flavoured vinegar to cover them completely. For a stronger vinegar, you can strain off the vinegar and pour it over a fresh lot of herbs half-way through.

Popular herb vinegars are: Basil, lovely with Tomato salads; Dill, which you can use in sauces for fish; Tarragon, which has a light summery smell; Chervil; Sage; Thyme; Rosemary; Burnet, which has a lovely affinity with Cucumber; or Mint. Elderflowers make an unusual vinegar. You can also use seeds – Dill, Fennel and Celery, for example.

SPICES

Exotic spices came to Europe from south China and the East Indies, along ancient trade-routes. They were shipped from the Eastern Mediterranean to Genoa or Venice, for distribution through Northern Europe. For centuries bloody wars were fought over the spice trade, as Venetians, Genoese, Dutch, English and Portuguese battled for control of the trade routes for these lucrative commodities.

There is evidence of English spice-use as early as the Bronze Age. But it was the Romans who first set up regular supply-lines: their cooks could not function without spices. After the Romans pulled out, occasional supplies may have arrived with Phoenician traders; there are words for Ginger in both Anglo-Saxon and Middle-English.

Once the Norman Conquest opened Britain to French influence, spice-consumption soared. Thereafter English cookery continued to rely on a steady demand of spices until well into the eighteenth century. There was a hiccup in the mid-seventeenth when the Puritans, those foes of fleshly pleasure, forbade the use of spices and rich, elaborate dishes in general. As reaction, Restoration foodies put lots of spices into their wonderfully rich cookery.

Fierce competition and the opening up of new fast sea routes to the Far East, however, gradually brought spice prices down. As they became cheap and popular, their status among the wealthy, and their use in *haute cuisine* declined.

Insatiable Western demand for aromatic spices came not only from cooks – Ginger and Cinnamon in particular were also highly valued as drugs. Both the Greeks and the Romans were quick to appreciate the digestive first aid that the aromatic spices could offer. The cookery books of Apicius – of which it has been said that they describe 'the delicious meals eaten across civilized Europe during the centuries of Roman domination' – feature spices at every turn. John Edwards, who translated and adapted this ancient culinary best-seller as *The Roman Cookery of Apicius* has calculated that over 90 per cent of the 500 recipes it contains called for costly imported spices.

One of Apicius' basic recipes is for Spiced Salts, ordinary salt to which over half its weight in Pepper, Ginger, Cumin and other herbs and spices was added. 'Spiced salts', notes Apicius, 'are good for the digestion, for promoting regularity, and for averting all sorts of sickness and plagues and chills.'

Medieval cooks may have used spices in much the same way: to ease the digestive burden of the enormous meals served up at the rich man's table, in which flesh, fowl and fish were eaten to unhealthy excess. Certainly many Medieval physicians were aware that their rich patients' diet was seldom a very healthy one. Francesco Di Marco Datini, a wealthy and rather greedy fourteenth-century merchant of Prato, in Northern Italy, was always having moderation at table preached at him by his physician. He suggested that Datini throw away all physic exept for Cassia, a popular purge; to use it only when strictly necessary – 'and then use it with Ginger', and that he eat a little Ginger jam before dinner, to encourage urination.

By the eighteenth century, however, the use of herbs and spices as medicine was beginning its gradual decline in English use, ousted by the new chemical medicines. By the early twentieth century, spices such as Ginger and Cinnamon lingered on in the *British Pharmacopoeia* only in minor roles; Ginger was an ingredient, for instance, of Peacock's Stomachic Mixture, warmly recommended for flatulence.

In our own time, however, when bland and sweet seem to have become the prevailing tastes in Western food, the highly spiced cookery of the Middle East, India, and China has powerful new appeal. Just as we turn to Morocco or India for instruction in the gastronomic use of spices, so we go East to learn the full spectrum of talents concentrated in these wonderful food-medicines. In Chinese and Indian cookery, small amounts of Ginger are added to almost every recipe for meat or fish, to stimulate your taste-buds, improve your digestion, and help your intestines detoxify flesh or fish.

Medicine or gastronomy? Happily, there is no need to make a distinction.

And Ezechias rejoiced at their coming, and he shewed them the storehouse of his aromatical spices, and of the silver, and of the gold, and of the sweet odours, and of the precious ointment, and all the storehouses of his furniture, and all things that were found in his treasures.
Isaias, Chap XXXIX v.2

BLACK PEPPER

In the tropical forests of Asia, Peppers grow in long strings of berries, which ripen from green to bright vermilion. The green berries are dried to make black Pepper; the ripe ones to make the slightly milder white Pepper which purists prefer for paler-coloured dishes.

Pepper came West in classic times, and rapidly became the most popular spice of them all. Roman cooks sprinkled it freely on almost every dish. The Goths and Vandals soon acquired a taste for it. Western Europe soon found it quite as indispensable, and the ports of the Levant and the Adriatic fattened on the trade.

We think of Pepper as a spice to use with savoury dishes. In fact it can be intriguing with sweet or fruity tastes. Hardy Amies, that noted gourmet, once persuaded me to try it with a beautiful ripe strawberry – unusual and delicious.

Black Pepper is considered one of the great tonics in Chinese medicine, stimulating and energizing in 'cold' problems such as 'flu, coughs and poor circulation.

In her marvellous book *The Herbs of Life*, US herbalist Lesley Tierra gives a recipe for Chai Tea, which she says is drunk all over India as a spicy, stimulating winter beverage – good preventative medicine.

To make: combine 1 ounce fresh grated Ginger, 7 Peppercorns, 1 Cinnamon stick, 5 Cloves, 15 Cardamom seeds and 1 Orange peel with 1 pint of water. Cover the pot, heat and simmer for 10 minutes. Add ½ cup milk and simmer another 10 minutes. Strain and sweeten with honey. It is usually made with black tea in India. However, for those who do not want to ingest the caffeine, make it with herbs alone.

CARAWAY

Caraway seed cake is an unfortunate introduction to this spice for many people. I hated the mouthfuls of spiky little seeds as a child, and have never liked the taste of Caraway since. But in northern Europe – which has made Caraway its own – it turns up all the time. It is particularly popular in Cabbage dishes, rescuing them from the windiness that overcooked Cabbage produces.

In Elizabethan times, Caraway was highly valued as a digestive herb, and little saucers of Caraway seeds were put on the table for people to nibble whenever baked Apples were served. For centuries more, it was popular in the form of Caraway comfits, a sweetmeat in which the tiny seeds received up to a dozen separate coatings of sugar syrup.

CARDAMOM

Cardamom belongs to the same family as Ginger, and the bushes grow wild in the Indian tropical jungles. Brought West in the long slow caravans of the spice trade, it has always been expensive, often faked or adulterated. *Never* buy it ground – look for the small, whole greenish pods.

A wonderful spice, Cardamom stimulates the mind and heart; it is said to promote clarity of thinking. In Ayurvedic medicine it is considered to be one of the best and safest of digestive stimulants. It is also claimed that it detoxifies the caffeine in coffee – one reason, perhaps, why a couple of pods of Cardamom are so often stuck in the spout of the silver Bedouin coffee pot. If you are a caffeine junkie, try the Cardamom treatment. The flavour of Cardamom is perfectly delicious; a travel-writer friend of mine, Angela Humphery, always adds a couple of pods to the ornate china pot of aromatic herb tea that replaces coffee on her dinner-table.

In traditional Eastern medicine, Cardamom is used to treat mucus congestion in the lungs. It is also believed to neutralize the mucus-forming quality of milk and fruit.

CAYENNE
OR
CHILLI PEPPERS

What Ginger is to Eastern medicine, Cayenne is to much of Western traditional medicine. The North American Indians made extensive use of it, a supreme tonic for the heart and circulation. Through a famous nineteenth century US herbalist called Samuel Thomson, it reached Britain to become a popular botanic remedy for every kind of fever and acute infection; in the back street slums of Britain's dark industrial cities, there was plenty of infectious disease. The botanic practitioners who worked in these slums administered Cayenne as a first-resort remedy in all such cases – huge doses of as much as a teaspoon of the raw powder – that had regular doctors branding them reckless quacks and murderers. Yet Cayenne often worked miracles in such cases, thanks to its supreme tonic and disinfectant powers.

Today Cayenne is attracting the attention of cardiac specialists, because of its apparent ability to dissolve clots in the bloodstream.

We can be sure from Bertie Wooster's description that a massive dose of Cayenne was the wonder ingredient in Jeeves' miracle morning-after reviver.

US herbalist Dian Dincin Buchman, who describes Cayenne as one of her favourite herbs, often exploits this stimulating property. On long drives, she keeps a thermos of grape juice laced with Cayenne in the glove compartment, to give her a boost when she starts to feel jaded.

Cayenne is also a powerful antiseptic, and Mexican Indians are among the native peoples who have relied on it to detoxify doubtful foods, sprinkling it freely over savoury dishes.

Cayenne is an acquired taste. The slightest hint will send some people screaming to the fridge for ice, whereas a Pakistani friend of ours will sit at table chewing Chilli Peppers as a relish while he waits for dinner to be served. The children of that lovely eccentric herbalist Juliette de Baïracli Levy got used to the taste young.

I was able to risk raw milk daily for (them) . . . even from cows and goats of uncertain health, as I cut half a pod of cayenne into every cup of milk and let it steep. This I knew would destroy harmful bacteria. The pepper gave the milk a hot biting taste, but my children learnt to take it with pleasure.

Presently he came back with a glass on a tray.

'If you would drink this, sir,' he said, with a kind of bedside manner, rather like the royal doctor shotting the bracer into the sick prince. 'It is a little preparation of my own invention. It is the Worcester Sauce that gives it its colour. The raw egg makes it nutritious. The red pepper gives it its bite. Gentlemen have told me they have found it extremely invigorating after a late evening.'

I would have clutched at anything that looked like a life-line that morning. I swallowed the stuff. For a moment I felt as if somebody had touched off a bomb inside the old bean and was strolling down my throat with a lighted torch, and then everything seemed suddenly to get all right. The sun shone in through the window; birds twittered in the tree-tops; and, generally speaking, hope dawned once more.

Carry On, Jeeves
(P. G. Wodehouse, 1925)

Eaten raw in these ways, Cayenne is much milder than when cooked, when it develops its fiercest bite. If you burn your mouth or throat with a red-hot curry, sip beer, wine or milk: the fiery chemicals that give Chillis their bite dissolve in fat or alcohol.

CINNAMON
One of the most highly esteemed warming and stimulating herbs of traditional Chinese medicine, Cinnamon is prescribed to raise vitality, stimulate the circulation, and help clear congestion of every kind: just the thing for winter.

An early French herbal, *Le Livre des Simples*, recommended it for 'weakness of the stomach and liver and to help digestion weakened by cold . . .'. Those who think of Cinnamon as a mild pudding sort of a herb, however, will be surprised to learn that it is also one of the most powerful antiseptics. In times of plague, people used to go around wearing little pierced wooden boxes filled with herbs they hoped would protect them – the most important ingredient being Cinnamon. Numbers of people – Elizabeth David and myself among them – were put off Cinnamon by being dosed with it at boarding school to ward off colds or 'flu. At the beginning of this century, in fact, the Cinnamon Treatment (see p.150) was recognized as a reliable cure for 'flu in its earliest stages.

In the Far East, Cinnamon is an indispensable ingredient of curry powders, and pilau rice. In cooler Western Europe, it is the warming qualities of Cinnamon that are particularly appreciated, in traditional recipes like Hippocras and Mulled Wine, and added to stewed fruit, or milk puddings. It has a particular affinity with Apples. Cinnamon toast was until recently a popular tea-time treat, made by sprinkling brown sugar and powdered Cinnamon on hot buttered toast.

For a warming winter drink, try Cinnamon Milk. Add a stick of Cinnamon to a small panful of milk; bring it to the boil, then simmer over very low heat for 5-10 minutes. Add a teaspoon of honey to each cupful.

CLOVES

Cloves are the dried flower-buds of a little grey-leaved evergreen tree, native to the Molucca Islands in the South Philippines. For centuries, Cloves were the most expensive of all spices and prized accordingly; the home-grown substitute was the Clove-Gilly flower

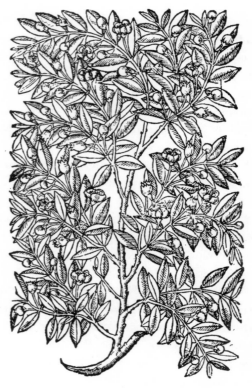

or Dianthus, so-called because its petals infused in wine gave a pleasantly spicy taste.

Cloves are powerful medicine, a general stimulant and a mental tonic too; St Hildegarde of Bingen thought highly of Cloves, and recommended them for headaches, migraine and deafness after a cold – presumably due to sinus congestion. Cloves are good for the digestion, too, and they can help counter nausea. Like Cinnamon, Cloves were long valued for their antiseptic powers, and an Orange stuck all over with Cloves was an up-market insurance against the Plague. In fact, modern aromatherapy research has vindicated this claim: a 1 per cent emulsion of Clove has an antiseptic strength 3-4 times greater than the carbolic acid with which Lister revolutionized surgery.

Wonderfully warming, Cloves will help you sail through winter with never a cough or cold. Add a bruised clove or two to a cupful of

Camomile tea or a hot Lemon and honey, whenever you feel chilly.

Bread sauce, with its preparatory infusion of Cloves, Onions and a Bayleaf in milk, is a last trace of an earlier and more adventurous use. Made properly, it is even more delicious than the chicken, turkey or pheasant it is meant to accompany.

CORIANDER

Coriander was brought to Britain from the Mediterranean by the Romans, and in the Middle Ages it was grown by every self-respecting gardener or housewife. Medieval cooks loved it with meat, particularly pork. Unlike most of the aromatic spices, Coriander has always been considered a cooling spice, used to offset the bite and pungency of hot spices such as Chilli.

In the far East, Coriander is prescribed for both digestive problems such as griping stomach pains, and for urinary tract infections.

It also has an agreeable pep-up action, as a 'euphorizing' spice – good for when you are feeling low or rundown.

Today Coriander is being produced in Britain in huge quantities, as the immigrant market and our growing taste for exotic flavours has produced a demand not only for the seed, but also for the parsley-like leaves with the odd and to many people, disagreeable smell.

In pre-refrigeration days, Coriander was used as a preservative: the Romans mixed it with Cumin and vinegar and rubbed it into meat to keep it sweet and fresh.

The Greeks use it extensively; mushrooms and other vegetables cooked à la Grecque have been simmered in a mix of Olive oil, white wine or vinegar, Peppercorns, a Bayleaf and plenty of Coriander seeds. It is a taste with a great affinity for pork; the Pork Afelia that is a stock item on every Greek restaurant menu is strongly seasoned with Coriander.

King Richard II's cooks loved the combination too, and used it for an aromatic marinade called Cormarye, in which Coriander, Caraway, Peppercorns and crushed Garlic were pounded together and added to red wine, which was used to cover and baste a loin of pork. Just delicious!

SEED WATER
Take a Spoonful of Coriander Seed, half a Spoonful of Caraway-Seed bruised, and boild in a Pint of Water, then strain it, and bruise it up with the Yolk of an Egg, and so mix it with Sack and double refined Sugar, according to your Palate.

The Art of Cookery
Made Plain and Easy
(Hannah Glasse, 1747)

CUMIN

Cumin is a hot-climate plant with pretty little mauve-white flowers, closely related to Fennel and Coriander; the Romans loved it so much for flavouring that they worked hard at growing it even in the chilly British Isles. Medieval gardeners followed suit.

The cookery of the Middle East is unthinkable without the deep, sweet pungent note of Cumin. And when you wander past the wonderful spice stalls in a North African market, it is the dizzying smell of Cumin that you notice most.

Cumin is yet another friend to the digestive system, and a tonic to the heart and nervous system too.

When you use Cumin in cookery, the seeds should be warmed first to help release their flavour. Toss them over a low fire in a heavy pan for a couple of minutes.

Cumin is diuretic, it eases and disperses flatulence. In food, sauces or stews, it helps digestion. Item, the wine in which it has been cooked with fennel seed takes away stomach and intestinal pain caused by flatulence.

Le Livre des Simples

GINGER

In the traditional medicine of China, and the Ayurveda of India – systems developed centuries before the birth of Christ – Ginger had a place of high honour, a food-medicine with an unequalled range of uses. Ayurvedic doctors call Ginger 'the universal medicine'; widely used for digestive and respiratory diseases, a tonic to the heart, a boon to the arthritic; applied topically, it is also a wonderful pain-killer.

In Chinese and Indian cookery, small amounts of Ginger are added to almost every recipe for meat or fish, to stimulate the taste-buds, improve the digestion and help the intestines detoxify flesh or fish.

It has been estimated that at least half the herbal prescriptions written by traditional Chinese doctors contain a little Ginger. It may be acting as a catalyst, to boost the assimilation and efficacy of the chief herbs in the formula; it may counter cramps or painful spasms if the main herbs could produce this effect. Or it may be included to add a little warmth when the chief herbs have a markedly cooling effect. (The English custom of sprinkling a little ginger over melon, a particularly 'cooling' food, is an echo of this approach.)

By the first century AD, Ginger was already a familiar drug to physicians of the Middle East and southern Europe; in the first Western herbal, Dioscorides' *De Materia Medica*, Ginger is described as particularly useful to the digestion – a relaxant for the stomach.

The *Regimen Sanitatis*, a long medical treatise written *c* the eleventh century, was read and quoted extensively throughout Europe during much of the Medieval period; it praised Ginger as both prevention and cure, excellent for weak stomachs.

'Ginger', wrote John Gerard in his famous seventeenth-century *Herbal*, ' . . . is right good with meat in sauces, or otherwise in conditures; for it is of an heating and digesting qualitie, and is profitable for the stomacke . . . '.

By the nineteenth century much of the Ginger imported to England was being used in the manufacture of sharp, strongly-flavoured

---

CONNYNGES IN CYRIP
Take connynges and seth hem wel in gode broth. Take wyne greke, and do thereto with a porcion of vynegar and floer of canell, hoole clowes, quybibes hoole, and oother gode spices, with raisons, coraunce and gyngyn ypared and ymynced. Take up the connynges and smyte hem on pecys, and cast hem into the siryppe and seeth hem a litel on the fyre and serve it forth.

The Forme of Cury
N.B. This is a recipe from the Court cooks of King Richard II. Greek wine was sweet, and the addition of Raisins, Currants, Cinnamon, Cloves, Cubebs, and peeled minced Ginger would have produced a dense, rich, aromatic syrup – a striking foil for the somewhat dry, bland, flesh of rabbits. Such sweet-sour and aromatic combinations of flavours were delightful to the Medieval palate.

made-up sauces, curry powders and Ginger pop or beer. In household cooking, it was confined to cakes, to puddings like that wonderful nursery treat Steamed Ginger Pudding, to local specialities such as parkin and Gingerbread, and to home-made wines and beers.

Until fairly recently, most British shoppers knew Ginger only in pale powder form. Within the last few years the fresh whole tubers of Ginger have become widely available in supermarkets as well as ethnic shops, thanks to heavy demand from immigrants, together with the soaring popularity of both Chinese and Indian cooking. Neither is possible without lavish supplies of fresh Ginger.

NUTMEG

The Nutmeg is the kernel of the fruit of the Nutmeg tree; the bright scarlet flesh dries to a brownish-yellow to supply another very similar spice – Mace.

Like most of the spices, Nutmegs are warming, and a fillip to the digestive system. They are also considered calming to the nerves; overdose on them, however, and the effect could be just the opposite – giddiness and stupefaction.

When I was a child, junket was often served as a pudding. I liked the sweet pink kind, but much preferred the creamy-white plain junket, with its delicate speckling of Nutmeg.

Although not a pushy, aggressive spice, once you get used to Nutmeg with any food, the same dish tastes bland and boring without it. The Dutch seldom serve cool, green winter vegetables – particularly Spinach, Cabbage and Cauliflower – without a liberal seasoning of Nutmeg; I picked up this habit from my Dutch husband.

Nutmeg is one of the two spices which make this eighteenth-century recipe for Apple fritters deliciously different.

TO MAKE FINE FRITTER

Put to half a Pint of thick Cream four Eggs well beaten, a little Brandy, some Nutmeg, and Ginger, make this into thick Batter with Flour, and your Apples must be Golden Pippins, pared and chopped with a Knife; mix all together, and fry them in Batter. At any time you may make an alteration in the Fritters with currants.

> The Art of Cookery
> Made Plain and Easy
> *(Hannah Glasse, 1747)*

TURMERIC

When you enjoy that livid yellow pickle called Piccalilli, you are eating Turmeric, which is where the yellow comes from. You may be eating it in cheap mustard too – it is a classic way to fake mustard. To many people – myself among them until recently – that sums up Turmeric: the poor man's Saffron, a cheap way to turn dishes bright yellow. My eyes were opened when I talked to a group of Indian women after a herbal lecture, as I mention in the Foreword.

In Indian traditional medicine, Turmeric is valued as a blood purifier, an excellent natural antibiotic, and a tonic to the metabolism. It is used to regulate the menstrual cycle and relieve cramps, to reduce fevers, improve poor circulation and to help sort out skin disorders. As first aid, it is used for boils, burns, sprains, swelling and bruises.

Turmeric is often taken as a remedy in the form of a milk decoction; make it like Cinnamon Milk, above, p.38. It is also often taken as a tea. The powder can be mixed with water or honey to make a paste for external application.

WILD FOOD

When a countrywoman in the past wanted something different for a salad, some healthy green leaves to boil up with the bacon, or fruit to make into jams, jellies, wines or puddings, she raided the vast free larder of the countryside.

At different times of the year her harvest might include: Nettles; Dandelion leaves; Sorrel; Bistort; Hawthorn buds; Alexanders; Ramsons; Chickweed; Fat Hen; Orache; Mallows; Wild Beets; white or black Mustards; Horseradish roots; Scurvygrass; and Watercress. The berries and fruits would include Blackberry and Dewberry; wild Strawberries; Bilberries; Hips and Haws; Crab-Apples; Sloes; Elderberries; Bullace Plums; and Rowanberries. For diets short of good protein, there were always nuts – Beech and Hazelnuts, Sweet Chestnuts and Walnuts. For homemade wines, there were Cowslips, Elderflowers, Primroses, Oak leaves, Coltsfoot, Hawthorn blossoms.

In Chinese medicine, wild foods are believed to have tonic qualities quite apart from their intrinsic nutritional value, because of their ability to adapt to their natural environment. 'Herbs that have adapted themselves to grow in harsh, rugged environments tend to impart their acquired strength to one who uses them,' says Michael Tierra.

At times of national want or emergency, we remember these hedgerow riches; during the 1939-45 war, parties of schoolchildren, Boy Scouts and Girl Guides were sent out to harvest Hips and Haws, a rich source of the vitamin C no longer imported in the shape of Oranges. Little guidebooks to these wild foodstuffs were published, together with Hints from the Ministry of Food. After the war, however, we slipped back into our former ignorant ways. Most of us could not identify half of these plants today; do *you* know what Alexanders look like?

Some of the plants are practically endangered species, if they have not already disappeared; when did you last see a field yellow with Cowslips? In much of England, the kind of countryside you can stroll through is shrinking by the day, to be replaced with vast prairies of crops, bordered by thin strips of muddy land or a main road. Many of the remaining hedgerows are alongside country roads, where they are exposed to the lead-laden exhaust gases of passing cars, or routinely 'controlled' with doses of weedkiller by zealous local Councils.

Many of the most valuable and tasty of edible wild plants, however, are those which are most abundant, sprouting lavishly on derelict land, on commons or open heath and moor, or in wild woodland. On open parkland in or near big cities, we are often understandably barred from harvesting the wild plants that make them so attractive. But out in the countryside, in odd corners of land in cities, even in your own back garden, you will find plenty of wild food ready and waiting. A few Nettles or Dandelion leaves, the odd Elder blossom or bouquet of Mayflowers, a handful of Ramsons leaves or the bagful of Blackberries will not be missed.

Harvest wild foods well away from farm crops, where they might get dowsed with pesticide sprays, or from road verges where they could be contaminated by passing traffic.

Apart from the fact that they cost you nothing, wild foods have one more great advantage over most shop-bought fruit and vegetables: they are all organically grown.

The wild food plants in this section are the commonest of country fare. If you become more adventurous, or more curious, there are excellent books showing exactly what you can harvest – and how to distinguish the edible from the poisonous.

All plants are now protected by law, and you are breaking the law if you uproot plants without permission from the owner of the land where they are growing. A number of plants are now endangered species, and it is forbidden to harvest them at all.

As a general rule, only harvest plants and weeds which are particularly abundant, like those mentioned in this chapter.

LEAVES

CHICKWEED

People go to great trouble rooting Chickweed out of their gardens, yet according to Juliette de Baïracli Levy, this insignificant creeping herb, too weak even to stand upright, 'is one of the supreme healers of the herbal world, and has given me wonderful results.' She recommends it enthusiastically as soothing and healing for the digestive tract, the bowels and the lungs.

Chickweed remains green almost the whole year round, but if you intend to put it in a salad, it should be picked in early summer, before the leaves turn stringy. Chickweed leaves have a mild unobtrusive flavour; combine them with sharper-tasting greens such as Watercress or Rocket, with plenty of Garlic in the dressing. It is claimed that they taste like Spinach when cooked; Euell Gibbons, who sampled Chickweed cooked in a number of different ways, found the flavour a little too unassuming for his taste; he suggests cooking it with other greens, adding it about 2 minutes

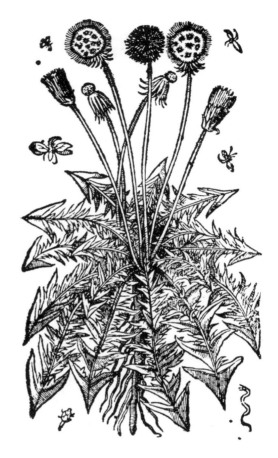

before the end of the cooking time.

Like all the edible wild green leaves, Chickweed can also be added – as the Medieval peasant did – to thick green soups.

DANDELIONS

'A course of Dandelion treatment in the spring will tone up your whole body,' writes Jean Palaiseul, 'cleansing it of the waste matter deposited by the heavy clogging food of winter.' Rich in iron, Dandelion leaves are also a tonic for the blood and liver; a famous diuretic, they help get rid of excess cholesterol, and people with rheumatic or skin complaints should eat plenty of them. They also make one of the most delicious salads invented by the clever French, a wonderful contrast between the sharp clean taste of the leaves and the bland rich taste of the bacon; do try it.

Dandelion leaves can be cooked and *puréed* just like Spinach, or the leaves added to soups.

Salade de Pissenlit

Choose healthy young Dandelion leaves, wash them carefully, and put them in a salad bowl. Chop a few rashers of bacon into small pieces, heat a little oil in a pan, add the bacon and fry till crisp. Then add a tablespoon of white wine or white wine vinegar to the pan, heat up, and while it is still smoking, pour very quickly over the Dandelion leaves. Some chopped Onion or Garlic can be fried in the pan with the bacon.

HAWTHORN

Young Hawthorn leaves and buds used to be chewed by country children when they felt peckish; they were nicknamed Bread and Cheese. In the Cotswolds we called them Bread and Butter, and used to nibble them as we searched along the hedges for the sharp strong-looking thorns, which we needed for our old-fashioned gramophone.

Hawthorn buds are still used in parts of the country to make a savoury suet pudding; the light suet crust is rolled out long and thin, its surface then dotted with the green buds and very thin strips of bacon rashers. The pudding is rolled up, sealed and steamed for an hour or longer.

The green buds can also be added to salads; try them with a new Potato salad, dressed while the Potatoes are still warm with a light oil and vinegar dressing and plenty of snipped chives.

NETTLES

St Hildegarde of Bingen thought highly of Nettles: 'When [they] grow fresh out of the earth they are useful cooked as food for human beings because they purify the stomach and rid it of excess mucus or phlegm.' A modern herbalist would agree, adding that Nettles are also valuable for the anaemic and the rundown, for those with rheumatism and arthritis, and for those with digestive or skin problems.

Nettles are another of the great spring-cleaners, and spring is when they should be eaten, while the leaves are still tender. Only the tops should be gathered.

Pick, wash and dry a pint potful of Nettles and put them in a pint of salt water. (Bring to the boil), stir well and cook for 10 minutes. Melt 1 oz of bacon fat, stir in 1 oz of flour, add the nettles and water, and cook for another 5 minutes slowly, stirring all the time. Add a little boiling milk, and serve with croutons.

They Can't Ration These
(Vicomte de Mauduit, 1940)

As well as being valuable cleansers, Nettles are rich in vital nutrients, among them vitamins A and C, mineral salts including iron, calcium and potassium, and lots of chlorophyll. These riches become obvious when Nettles are fed to cattle or poultry; horses have lovely shiny coats and cows give richer milk.

Nettles obviously need to be cooked. Make a purée of them as a change from Spinach. Wash a big pile of them carefully, as you do with Spinach. Put them in a big pan, pressing them down with a spoon, add a couple of tablespoons of water, cover, and cook over low heat until they have melted down into a green mass. Drain them – keep the rich juice for soups – purée them in a blender together with a little seasoning, some butter and a grating of Nutmeg. Gourmets can add a couple of tablespoons of cream. In Scotland, Nettles are also made into a delicious pudding. **N.B.** Eat Nettles only once a week.

NETTLE PUDDING

Take 1 gallon of young Nettle-tops, thoroughly washed, add 2 good-sized Leeks or Onions, 2 heads of Broccoli or small Cabbage, or Brussels sprouts, and ¼lb of Rice. Clean the vegetables well, chop the Broccoli and Leek and mix with the Nettles. Place all together in a muslin bag, alternately with the Rice, and tie tightly. Boil in salted water, long enough to cook the vegetables, the time varying according to the tenderness or otherwise of the greens. Serve with gravy or melted butter.

A Modern Herbal
(Mrs M. Grieve, 1931)

This pudding was sometimes made with Oatmeal instead of Rice. If you use brown Rice instead of white, it should be cooked first or the greens will be sodden by the time the rice is cooked through. Nowadays we should steam the pudding in a basin tied up with a cloth, to prevent the goodness of the greens leaking away into the cooking water.

RAMSONS

Walking through coastal woodland with friends in Wales, I thought I spotted a bank of Snowdrops ahead. As we got nearer, though, a wonderful whiff of Garlic came breezing to our nostrils; it was Ramsons or Bear's Garlic, a cousin of the famous bulb, which is partial to damp woodland. Ramson leaves look like Lily of the Valley; if you harvest them young, while the starry white flowers are blooming from April to June, they add a mild Garlic flavour to your salads.

Ramsons are a country tonic for the heart and arteries, and will help protect you from strokes. They have a high sulphur content, making them excellent cleansers for the skin and for the bronchial tubes.

FRUITS AND BERRIES

BILBERRIES

In my childhood I once spent a memorable holiday in the Quantocks in Somerset. One fine afternoon we were taken Whortleberrying in the heath-covered hills. It was back-breaking work hunting out the little clouded dark blue berries, and their sharp taste was not enjoyable enough to make the job a pleasure. But at the end of the afternoon, when we had laboriously filled several baskets, we took them to a greengrocer shop in the neighbouring town; we were paid – lavishly we thought – for our toils.

Harvesting Whortleberries, or Bilberries as they are commonly called, is so labour-intensive that they have become an unattractive economic proposition. If you see them in shops, they are usually luxury items at high prices, often imported. If you find them wild, however, harvest and make the most of them.

An essential item in the currently popular Forest Fruits combinations beloved of yogurt-makers, they are also a sharp, deliciously different taste in fruits. Try them stewed in spiced red wine, or combined with Apples in a flan or a Charlotte (they have a great affinity for Apples).

Bilberries are a real treasury of herbal remedies. They are rich in fruit acids – malic, citric, benzoic – which paradoxically can help cleanse an over-acid system and help restore the alkaline reserve. Chew Bilberries if you have sores in your mouth or on your tongue, or a sore throat. They are powerfully antiseptic too; the Bilberry cure has been known to sort out nasty bouts of enteritis, dysentery, and food poisoning. In studies at St Bartholomew's Hospital, Bilberry juice wiped out colonies of a variety of bacilli – including that of typhoid – within 24 hours. Their leaves are also useful medicinally (see The Digestive System).

People suffering from night blindness should eat bilberries; the deep pigment helps regenerate the visual purple responsible for night vision.

Bilberry Jam

3lb of the fresh ripe fruit, and 1½lbs sugar; Bilberries need much less sugar for jam than most fruits. Clean the fruit and put it in a pan with the sugar and a cup of Apple juice. Bring to the boil, and boil briskly for 40 minutes. Bottle hot in screw-top jars.

A spoonful of this, held in the mouth then swallowed very slowly, will help a sore throat or painful sores in the mouth. For gut infections, put a spoonful in a glass of warm water, and take it 3-4 times a day.

BLACKBERRIES

Blackberrying is one of autumn's great pleasures – grown-ups enjoy it just as much as children. Blackberry and Apple tarts, Blackberry jam and thick Blackberry jelly can be the delicious rewards of the industrious picker. Blackberry cordial, made with the berries mixed with Cider, is still a popular country drink. Blackberry vinegar, another favourite for flavouring off-beat salads, is an excellent remedy for sore mouths or a touch of diarrhoea. For sore throats and hoarseness, a tablespoon of Blackberry jam can be sucked and swallowed slowly; like the Bilberry, the Blackberry is astringent and antiseptic.

Blackberry Cordial

Press out the juice from ripe Blackberries, add 900g/2lb of sugar to each quart, and ¼ oz of Nutmegs and Cloves (grate the Nutmeg). Boil for a short time, cool and strain. When cold, add a little brandy before bottling.

Blackberry Vinegar

Wash 900g/2lb of Blackberries and remove the stalks. Put them in a casserole, and cover with 600ml/1 pint of Apple cider vinegar. Put them in a low oven for a couple of hours, to let the juice run. Then strain into a stainless steel or enamel pan, add 900g/2lb of sugar, bring to the boil, and simmer gently for 5 minutes. If any scum rises, skim it off. Then take the pan off the heat, allow the mixture to cool and put into clean screwtop jars.

Take a spoonful of this in a little water as a gargle, for sore mouths or throats. In winter, when a cold threatens, add a couple of spoonfuls to a glass of hot water, with Lemon and honey. On a hot day, Blackberry vinegar in water is refreshing and thirst-quenching; it is useful and pleasant medicine for those with fevers.

ELDERBERRIES

Millions of clusters of the tiny black berries with the red stalks hang unregarded in our hedgerows every autumn; perhaps at least the birds enjoy them. Yet Elderberries can be made into marvellous tarts, jams, sauces, and wines; mixed with other fruit, particularly Apples, they contribute a sharp distinctive note of their own. You should eat them only in small quantities, because they are a laxative.

If you come in thoroughly chilled on a winter's day, or if you feel the first shiver of a cold or 'flu, a spoonful of Elderberry Rob –

which apothecaries used to sell – in a glass of hot water, with Lemon and honey, will help sort you out by inducing a healthy sweat. Drink it wrapped up warm, and repeat the dose at bedtime.

Apothecaries also sold a spiced Elderberry syrup, in which Ginger and Cloves enhanced the warming effect and added an antiseptic quality.

Elderberry Syrup
Wash and destalk the ripe berries. Put 900g/2lb of them in a pan with a cupful of water, and simmer until they have given up most of their juice. Crush and strain the berries through a sieve, put the juice back in the pan with 5 cloves, an inch or so of fresh Ginger root grated, and 225g/½lb sugar. Simmer for another hour, then store in tightly sealed jars.

TEA-TIME

The English have always been tea-drinkers, but it was not always Tea from China and the far East that they drank.

Tea as we know it only arrived in this country in the mid-seventeenth century, brought by the Dutch East India Company; hideously expensive, it sold for £3.10s a lb, a price that would be exorbitant in today's money. Soon our own East India Company was importing it; by the end of the century imports had risen to 20,000lbs a year, while the price had fallen to a mere 20s a lb. By the end of the eighteenth century imports had rocketed to 20,000,000lbs a year, and Tea had become our national drink – an honoured position it has never lost.

Its stimulating caffeine makes Tea so agreeable – and so addictive. Brewed up in the familiar brown earthenware pot, standing about shrouded in a tea-cosy, or left to stew at the side of the fireplace till it is a strong orange-brown in colour, Tea can develop lethally high levels of caffeine; a water-soluble alkaloid that can give you the shakes and wreck your digestion.

This is how Tea *should* be made. Warm the pot, put in 1 level teaspoon of Tea for the pot, and 1 more for each breakfast cupful you want, and pour on freshly boiling water; let it infuse for only 3 minutes, and then strain it off into another warmed pot and cover with a tea-cosy. Made like this, the caffeine count will be at the lower end of the estimated range: 20mg-110mg per cup for black Tea; 10-50mg a cup for Oolong Tea; or less than 35mg per cup for Green Tea.

Tea has been a prized herb for thousands of years. The ancient Greeks drank it for asthma, colds and bronchitis. In Chinese Traditional medicine, Green Tea is appreciated for its digestive properties and its ability to assist the circulation. In Russia green Tea is used to treat dysentery.

When Tea first reached London, much of it was green, from China, and in England too it was promoted as a health-giving drink, excellent for the digestion and useful for slimmers. In the long run, however, it was the cheaper black Teas from India that the English took to their hearts, often shockingly adulterated or faked.

Both kinds of Tea are now coming under scientific scrutiny, and astonishing benefits are being claimed. The tannins in Tea, it is said, can help lower blood pressure and cholesterol levels, protect the arteries, inhibit bacteria and viruses, and neutralize cancer-causing agents. Green teas are twice as rich as black in a group of tannins called catechins, which act as anti-oxidants to combat cancer and slow the ageing process. Milk added to tea, incidentally, neutralizes much of the tannin activity, although it makes Tea less likely to cause digestive problems.

In the Macrobiotic diet, two less familiar versions of the Tea plant are regularly drunk. One is Bancha Tea, made from the older leaves of the Tea-bush, not harvested until fall; they are drier and darker, and lower in caffeine than ordinary Tea. Bancha Tea is considered stabilizing, and good for the digestion – practising Macrobiotics drink it all the time. Bancha stem tea, otherwise known as Kukicha, is made from the smaller twigs, and contains calcium and other minerals, but almost no caffeine. An alkalizing tea, it refreshes, strengthens, and counters fatigue.

If your caffeine tolerance is low, try switching from black to one of the many green Teas from time to time – Oolong or Gunpowder, for instance.

Another way to lower the caffeine rating is to blend a mild Tea such as China or Gunpowder with equal amounts of a herb tea. The Chinese often add a few highly-scented flower petals to Tea, to lend it their lingering perfume; Jasmine is a favourite. Try Rose or Violet petals, Elderflowers or the flowering tops of Rosemary. These flowery brews would be ruined by milk, but if you feel they need a little sweetening, add a touch of honey.

Instead of a waterlogged slice of Lemon, add just a thin curl of peel, or a leaf or two of Lemon Verbena. You could also add a few drops of Orange Flower Water to your green Tea.

A favourite nineteenth century English recipe combined equal parts of dried Raspberry leaves, and either Blackcurrant or Balm leaves, with China tea. Mix, and make like ordinary tea. In another recipe, freshly dried Blackcurrant and Mint leaves were combined with green Tea.

TEA-TIME
They made a good deal of camomile tea, which they drank freely to ward off colds, to soothe the nerves, and as a general tonic. A large jug of this was always prepared and stood ready for heating up after confinements. The horehound was used with honey in a preparation to be taken for sore throats and colds on the chest. Peppermint tea was made rather as a luxury than a medicine; it was brought out on special occasions and drunk from wine-glasses. . . .

Lark Rise to Candleford
(Flora Thompson)

On a hot summer's day, try this Tea Frappé, not unlike an Italian *granita*.

Pour 900ml/1½ pints of boiling water over 4 tsp of China Tea. Strain it off after 5 minutes, let it cool and add 4 tsp of sugar and 2tbsp of freshly squeezed Lemon juice. Freeze to a mush. Serve with a sprig of Mint.

Whatever the benefits of Tea green or black, however, many people find by experience that they are better off without it – or at least with no more than a cup or two a day at most.

As a substitute for that indispensable cuppa, there are many herb teas to choose from. If you are lucky enough to have a garden, with its own corner for herbs, you may be growing some of them already. Many of the most healthy and delicious are already available in teabag form, among them Fennel, Chamomile, Rosehip, Hibiscus, Peppermint and Limeflower. Experiment to find one that you really enjoy. Once you have identified a couple of favourites, buy the dried herbs loose; the quantities in teabags are usually quite small. Better still, grow the herb yourself; most nursery gardens have a wide range these days, and others are available by post (see Useful Addresses, p.158). Teas made from fresh herbs often taste better, and are better medicine, than tea made from dried herbs. Whether in plant or dried form, try to get hold of herbs that have been organically grown.

A herbal infusion is excellent food-medicine, so suit your tea to your personal health needs: most of us are conscious of a weakness somewhere in our constitution. It may be your lungs or a weak circulation; a digestive system which occasionally lets you down; or skin that could be brighter and clearer.

Herb teas should never be drunk red-hot (nor indeed should any liquid at all); and they are most effective medicinally if they are sipped slowly.

There are numerous ways in which you can vary the flavour of your herbal tea. To enhance its digestive effect, you can bruise a Clove or a scrap of Cinnamon stick and infuse it with the tea. In winter add a shot of Apple juice to the water you make it with; or a scrap of dried Orange peel, a dried Liquorice stick, or a teaspoonful of Anise seeds (which will give it a delicious, warming taste rather like Liquorice). In summer, chill it and add a little Pineapple juice. For sweetening, use honey instead of sugar, Maple syrup or concentrated Apple juice.

Blends of two, three or more herbs often produce teas with a more pronounced flavour and a more interesting taste than straight herbal infusions. Our local herbalist in Rome made up a number of blends for everyday

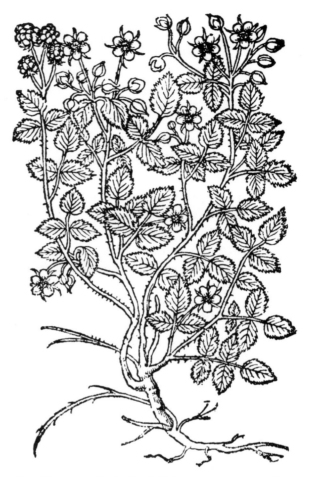

drinking; particularly delicious was a warming winter mix of Balm, Blackcurrant leaves, Peppermint and Anise seeds. Try experimenting.

Health-food shops – even supermarkets – sell dozens of ready-made herbal blends nowadays. Some of them are absolutely delicious, and others only passable. Others have had 'natural flavour' added to them, which to my mind can give them a slightly synthetic taste. I tend to shy away, too, from tea blends in which Spearmint figures prominently; all too often it is used to give a distinctive taste to a blend that might otherwise be fairly insipid.

Invest in a separate teapot for herbal teas – perhaps one of those stylish glass teapots, or a traditional china teapot used solely for herbal infusions. You may be making only a cupful at a time, but if you make it *in* a cup, it still has to be strained into another cup.

The following list of herbs that make good drinkable teas also tells you what they could be doing for your general health.

AGRIMONY

A tea made from the leaves and flowers of Agrimony was once widely drunk all over Northern Europe. It has an agreeable taste, and turns a pretty claret colour. An astringent, slightly bitter herb, it is good for kidney and urinary problems and diarrhoea; by the same token, if you have a tendency to constipation, you should avoid it. Use 1-2 teaspoons per cup, and let it infuse for 10-15 minutes.

BALM

Balm tea has a delicate lemony flavour, and was for centuries a popular English country tea. A tonic for mind and body, Balm was considered by Paracelsus – the sixteenth-century medical revolutionary – a great antidote to ageing and senility. Modern herbalists prescribe it for depression, digestive problems, menstrual cramps, and as a tonic for the heart; it is also a mild useful remedy for high blood pressure. Use a couple of teaspoons of the dried herb – more of the fresh – to a cupful of boiling water; infuse covered for 10-15 minutes. Balm is a good mixer, often used in the past to 'stretch' expensive ordinary Tea.

BETONY

Another popular everyday tea, '. . . the leaves and flowers by their sweet and spicy taste comfort both in meat and medicine', said Gerard. Betony was once considered a perfect panacea for any ills affecting the head; modern herbalists still consider it excellent for those suffering from nerves or stress. Infuse a teaspoon of the dried herb in a covered pot for 10-15 minutes.

BLACKCURRANT

The tea made from Blackcurrant leaves has a fresh and pleasant taste. Like Balm, the leaves are an excellent substitute for regular tea; in fact, in times gone by the poor used to eke out their precious supplies of Indian tea with Blackcurrant leaves. It is particularly refreshing in summer.

Modern French phytotherapists prescribe an infusion of Blackcurrant leaves to be taken regularly by their rheumatic and arthritic patients; it counters acidity and helps cleanse the system.

Use 2 teaspoons of the fresh leaves for every cup. Put them in a small pan with a cupful of water, bring gently to the boil, then take off the heat and infuse covered for 10 minutes. If you are using the dried leaves, soak them for an hour in cold water before making your infusion. To do this, pour a cupful of boiling water over 2 tsp dried herbs; infuse 10-15 minutes.

CATNIP

This was a favourite country tea long before the real thing arrived from the Far East, and it continued to be widely drunk for many years after. Its fans claimed that it did everything that ordinary Tea could do without the side-effects. A many-purpose herb, it is an excellent nerve-tonic; drink it hot at bedtime for sound sleep without nightmares. A useful cold and 'flu preventive, it is also a boon to disordered digestions.

CHAMOMILE

Perhaps the most widely-appreciated of all herbal infusions apart from Tea itself, Chamomile is an anti-spasmodic that has been used for centuries for convulsions, ague and colicky pain; it soothes the nerves and calms the digestion (but drink it *before* rather than after meals). It can help with a variety of menstrual problems, too. It also helps you to sleep. Chamomile is a good tea for the sickroom, especially for those with fever. Use a couple of teaspoons of the papery heads to a cupful of boiling water. Infuse covered for about 10 minutes.

ELDERFLOWER

This is another cooling summer tea, although more often used to ward off colds and 'flu, since it promotes a healthy perspiration. Infuse 1 of the whorls of creamy, sweet-smelling flowers in a pint of boiling water, covered, for 5-10 minutes. Strain. Elderflower is good drunk cold, too.

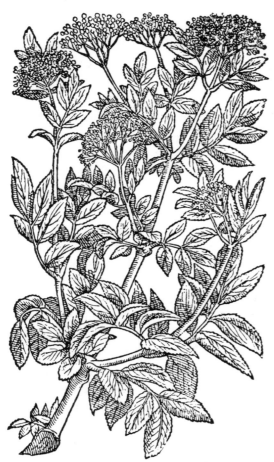

FENNEL

Tea made from the seeds of Fennel has a delicious spicy aroma, and sweetened with a little honey it is an excellent breakfast Tea. Good for weak windy digestive systems, for getting rid of excess phlegm in the lungs, it also damps down appetite (the Anglo-Saxons drank Fennel tea to help them through the hunger-pangs of Lent). Crush 1 teaspoon of the seeds per cup, and infuse covered for 10 minutes.

FENUGREEK

Another lovely spicy, aromatic tea, golden in colour. Fenugreek has a high reputation, especially in the Middle East, as a cleanser and expeller of excess mucus in the respiratory or digestive system. The little seeds are highly nutritious – eat them when you have drunk the Tea. To make, crush a teaspoon of the seeds, and simmer them covered for 5 minutes in a cupful of water.

HAWTHORN

The leaves of the Hawthorn were often used in the past to bulk out more interesting teas. They are one of the ingredients of a popular country Tea mix: 2 parts of dried Hawthorn leaves to 1 part each of Sage and Balm; or equal parts of Hawthorn, Sage, Balm and Blackcurrant leaves.

In German folk medicine, the leaves are valued as a heart tonic, along with the blossoms and the fruit. A tea is made from leaves and blossoms; use a heaped teaspoon to a cupful of boiling water, and let them infuse for 6 minutes. Austrian herbalist Maria Treben recommends Hawthorn Tea for poor circulation, headaches, lapses of memory, cardiac problems, and arteriosclerosis.

HIBISCUS FLOWERS

This tea looks very pretty, with its deep claret

colour, and tastes particularly refreshing on a hot day. However, it is also a good cooling Tea, good for mild fevers, or for drinking when you are particularly hot and thirsty. It is also useful for minor stomach complaints.

LIMEFLOWER

This gentle, mild-flavoured tea simply tastes nice. It has such a lot to offer, however, that it is deservedly one of the classic herbal teas, widely drunk all over Europe and available in teabag form even in supermarkets these days. Limeflowers are anti-spasmodic and sedative to the nerves and the digestive system. Drink it after meals as a *digestif*, and in the evening to help you unwind and relax. Victims of stress should drink it instead of their regular caffeine fix. Modern French research suggests that it may counter plaque formation in the blood – so drink it for your heart's sake, too. Use 1 teaspoon of the dried flowers to a cupful of boiling water, and infuse for 10 minutes.

PEPPERMINT

'A balm for the entire digestive tract,' says French herbalist Maurice Messegue; there is no finer *digestif* after a rich and heavy meal than a cupful of Peppermint tea. If you make it from the fresh plant growing on your own windowsill it will be better still, a beautiful, bright green brew. Peppermint tea will allay gripes, cramps and spasms, and calm nausea. A teaspoonful of dried leaves should be infused in a cupful of boiling water, covered; or use a tablespoon of the fresh leaves.
N.B. Like other members of the Labiatae family – Rosemary, Sage and Thyme – Peppermint Tea should not be drunk too often.

RED CLOVER

A tea made from Red Clover blossoms, has a mild, delicate flavour, and is slightly sweet. Use at least half a dozen of the fresh heads (1-3 teaspoons of the dried) to a cupful of boiling water; infuse covered for 5 minutes. Excellent for the skin problems of both adults and children, its calcium and phosphorus content makes it valuable for bones and teeth too. Its demulcent qualities make Red Clover a soothing drink for sufferers from acid indigestion, asthma and respiratory problems.

ROOIBOSCH

This is a godsend for those who are sensitive to caffeine, but do not feel that a mild herbal infusion is a decent substitute for their favourite cup of Tea. The leaves of this shrubby plant from South Africa are brewed just like tea-leaves – 1 teaspoon to a cupful of boiling water; you can add milk if you like. The smell is slightly offputting, but the taste is mild and extremely agreeable once you get used to it.

ROSEMARY

This tea is light, clean and fragrant. Drink it for breakfast to get you going at the start of a tough day. To make it, infuse 2-3 sprigs, covered, in a cupful of boiling water for 5 minutes.

SAGE

This tea is not everybody's cuppa: the pronounced flavour can be an acquired taste. But the Chinese, we are told, thought Sage tea infinitely preferable to the real thing they grew themselves, and were happy to receive boxes of Sage in exchange for chests of Tea. Sage is an excellent *digestif*; useful to help keep colds and 'flu at bay, and a tonic for convalescents. Do not make a habit of drinking Sage tea, however; have it only occasionally. To make it, pour a cupful of boiling water over 2-3 of the fresh or dried leaves, cover and infuse for 10 minutes.

BEAUTY
CARE

○

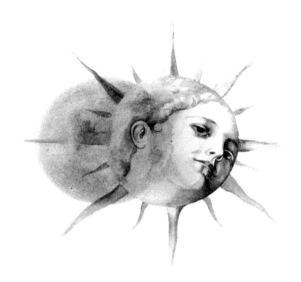

INTRODUCTION

For thousands of years, women all over the world have used plants to preserve and embellish their looks. Plants have supplied them with shampoo and hair conditioner; with creams to cleanse and soften their skins and lotions to tone them; with masques to revive them; with washes for sore or reddened eyes; with oils to perfume themselves, their surroundings or a fragrant bath; and with mild soaps for washing.

This herbal expertise was handed down over generations. As with the medicinal lore of plants, there was nothing fanciful or haphazard about it; plants were used for specific purposes, because they worked. And because they worked, their use became enshrined in centuries-long traditions.

Every Elizabethan housewife, for instance, knew that Cucumbers could soften and cool her skin; she pounded Lily roots to make a cream for sore or chapped skin; she brewed up Walnuts shells to make a rinse to darken her hair, or Chamomile flowers to lighten fair hair; she used a lotion made from the bright orange Marigolds in her garden to soothe and soften her skin, and extracts of Watercress to clear blemishes.

Such cosmetic traditions can be found all over the world, a fact shrewdly exploited by Anita Roddick of the Body Shop. Jojoba oil from the bean growing in Mexico and other hot countries is exceptionally resistant to oxidation; it has unique powers of penetrating and softening the skin, much more so than spermaceti oil from the sperm whale which it has largely replaced.

Aloe Vera is a clear gel from the thick greyish-green leaves of a cactus, renowned for its powers to soothe and heal. Pale green Henna powder from the dried shoots and leaves of the *Lawsonia alba* plant found in Africa and Asia has been used for thousands of years to dye hair, conditioning it to glossy softness at the same time. Hawaiian women have always used Cocoa butter to keep their skins soft and supple.

In the mid-twentieth century, such skin-care ingredients were being dismissed as old-fashioned. The future of cosmetic science, it was fondly believed, lay in the laboratory, where the new 'miracle' creams were being evolved.

The eclipse of plants was brief, however. By the 1970s, a new ecological awareness was growing, especially among women, who were beginning to question the wisdom of constantly applying synthetic chemicals to their skin. One after another, big cosmetic companies began cautiously experimenting with old-fashioned plants again.

This was quite often a policy decision, taken in the teeth of expert opinion. With no scientific literature to guide them, the cosmetic chemists of one big chain-store were forced to do their research in some unfamiliar places, 'from Culpeper right through to Mary Grieve and Potters *Cyclopedia*'. They talked to those who are using herbal extracts, conferring with Chelsea College Pharmacy department and the Institute of Science and Technology at the University of Wales. 'The perfume houses at Grasse in the South of France date back hundreds of years, and have tremendous knowledge.'

To make their final choice of herbs for use in a new skin-care range, the information they gleaned was fed into a computer, cross-referenced and the results studied. They were astonished to find the same plants coming up over and over again, for the same kind of use. The reaction of the human guinea-pigs who tested the range – supplied in plain plastic pots and bottles with simple typed labels – was another surprise, 'Quite staggering, the best we've ever had.'

Unlike England, France has never experienced a break in its traditions of herbal use; their cosmetic companies use plant extracts alongside more modern chemicals. The famous house of Clarins was launched in the 1950s with a range of pure, 100 per cent plant-extract oils for skin-care. Today, hundreds of plants are used in their ranges. Among them are Hazelnut oil to nourish and prevent moisture loss; Chamomile to soften and calm; Cypress to stimulate skin metabolism; Cornflower to refresh; Lime-flower to soothe and soften; Marjoram to re-vitalize; and Sage or Bilberry for their astringent qualities. Clarins – like the Body Shop – researches throughout the world, adding completely new plants to their range from time to time.

Cosmetic companies are now increasingly dependent on the world of plants, if only for shrewd commercial reasons; much of the research has been done for them already, over thousands of years, by countless women, and even the most brilliant findings can seldom be patented.

The science of skin-care is based on one fact: that the skin can be treated successfully from the outside, since it absorbs as well as excretes. This alone should make us wary of using skin-preparations containing man-made chemicals. Our skins are already ravaged by harsh sunlight, wind, cold; they suffer from poor diet, illness, stress, and the cumulative internal pollution of the synthetic chemicals we ingest along with what we eat and drink, and the air we breathe. It makes good sense not to increase our bodily load of pollution – for which our skins will pay – by the continuous application of more synthetic chemicals to our faces, hair, and bodies.

During a week-long fast – when one's senses, particularly that of smell, become very keen – I was surprised by my own reaction to two different skin-foods I had brought with me. Both were American; one of undeclared ingredients from a world-famous company, the other based on Jojoba and bee pollen, from a US range found only in health-food stores. After a few days fasting, I found the first began to have a harsh synthetic reek to it, to the point where I had to stop using it; the second smelled increasingly delicious.

When we use plant extracts on our skins we are using substances biologically compatible with our bodies, which they have no problem absorbing and assimilating. They can feed, tone, nourish, stimulate and revitalize far more effectively than any wonder-chemical.

It is said that you should put nothing on your face which you would not put into your mouth. Herbal cosmetic science goes further still; many of the herbs you put on your skin will work just as well from the inside as from the outside. Watercress, for instance, is a great blood-cleanser, high in antioxidants to help keep wrinkles at bay, and rich in blood-building chlorophyll, all helpful to your skin. Watercress used externally on the skin is excellent – as Culpeper pointed out – for a troubled skin.

If you are making a Chamomile or Lime-flower tisane at bedtime, use a couple of spoons as a calming and softening face wash. Carrot juice will improve your looks both drunk and applied to your skin. Many such uses are listed in the pages that follow. For busy women, it seems to me, these are eminently practical, time-saving ways to give our skin the benefits of herbs.

I am too lazy to start concocting my own creams, skin-potions and hair-conditioners, the more so since vegetable ingredients easily go off or become contaminated, unless you add just the right amount of the right preservatives. Without a garden where you can grow most of the plants you need, the problems of supply are daunting too. But if you are lucky enough to have a garden filled with fragrant flowers and herbs, making your own creams and lotions could be very rewarding; for some excellent books of practical advice and recipes see p.158.

Even if you cannot afford to buy skin-care products from the famous cosmetic houses increasingly using plant extracts, you will find plenty more reasonably-priced, plant-based ranges in your local health-food shop.

How do you know which product will work for you? Years ago, Countess Czaky, a brilliant Hungarian skin-care specialist, gave me some advice which I have never forgotten, and have found to be true: 'If a product does not suit your skin – your skin will know. It will soon tell you. And if it does – no matter how expensive the cream – stop using it straightaway.'

N.B. For ease of reference, herbs mentioned the first time in each treatment are in bold.

—————— BATHING BEAUTIES ——————

Ancient Egyptians, Greeks and Romans all loved bathing, and made a pleasurable, ceremonious therapy of it. But after the fall of the Roman Empire, the bath-less centuries descended on Europe; as late as the seventeenth century a bathroom was a rarity, particularly among the English.

Mary Stuart, wife of William of Orange and later Queen Mary II, doubtless learned cleaner ways during her brief years in Holland. Among the many improvements she made at Hampton Court with the assistance of Sir Christopher Wren, after her return to London, was to pull down the old Water Gallery and replace it with a suite of pretty little rooms for her own use, decorated with delicate wood carvings by Grinling Gibbons. One of these was a bathroom, with a splendid white marble bath, 'made very fine, suited either to hot or cold bathing as the season should invite'. It caused much talk.

Even in Regency times, a bathroom was still considered a luxury. It is a luxury I should find it extremely hard to do without. In times of stress or fatigue, or after a long day's overwork, there is nothing like the sensuous pleasure of a bath to revive jaded spirits. Simply soaking gently in hot water soothes and relaxes.

For true bathing-addicts, though, hot water is just the raw material. Any number of good things can be added to scent or soften it, to make it luxurious or therapeutic, a beauty treatment or a balm for shattered nerves.

I am not speaking of those vast plastic bottles of bubble bath, coloured in livid pinks, greens or yellows, rank with cheap synthetic perfumes, guaranteed to leave your skin bone-dry because of the strongly alkaline detergents they contain, which strip away the protective acid mantle of your skin. You can do better than that – and almost as cheaply. If you live in the country, or have your own garden, there is endless variety to enjoy. Even if you are a city-bound flat- or bedsit-dweller, the chemist, the supermarket and the health-food shop will

supply all you need for a wide range of beautifying or therapeutic baths.

Make your bathroom a pleasant refuge, as
appealing and pretty as possible, with a handy
shelf for books, drinks, bath essentials, and a
cassette player with your favourite tapes. Put
green plants in it – ferns are particularly at
home in the damp.

Avoid really hot baths; if you stagger out
with skin like a washerwoman, feeling drained
of life and energy, you have overdone it. Aim
for a bath that is pleasantly warm rather than
so hot that you can hardly put a toe in it
initially.

For a Bath *Take of Sage, Lavender
flowers, Rose flowers of each two handfuls,
a little salt, boil them in water or lye, and
make a bath not too hot in which bathe the
Body in a morning, or two hours before
Meat.*
The Receipt Book of John Middleton
(1734)

If you suffer from high blood pressure, or indeed any heart condition, or asthma, long hot
baths are not wise. They will not help varicose
veins, or cellulite, either. And unless you add
moisturizers to your bath, it will leave your
skin dried out. If you have just had a large
meal, forget the bath, too – it would be most
unkind to your digestion.

At the end of a hot bath, turn on the cold tap
and let the water cool down a little before you
get out. Or turn on the shower and give yourself a tepid-to-cool spray all over – cold if you
can bear it. Do not let your body get chilled,
however; wrap up warmly immediately afterwards and go straight to bed.

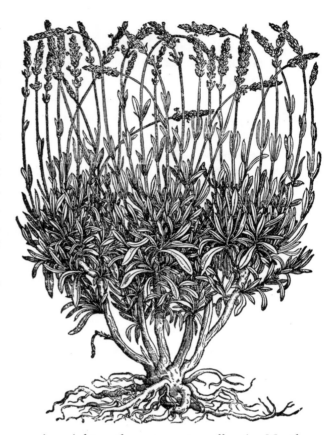

An eighteenth-century traveller in North
America noted that the Choctaw Indians used
'steam cabinets in which are boiled all sorts of
medicinal and sweet-smelling herbs. The
vapor filled with the essence and salts of these
herbs enters the patient's body through his
pores and his nose and restores his strength.'

The clever Choctaws knew a fact that we
are only just waking up to again – that whole,
hand- or foot-baths, like aromatherapy mas-
sages, are a wonderful way to exploit the healing properties of herbs, whether for specific
health problems or to improve the skin
through which they are absorbed. Some of
their healing powers will be absorbed directly
through the skin; others from the steam inhaled.

In your bathroom, you can be your own
herbalist.

Before you step into your bath, give your skin a quick toe-to-head brush with a special skin-brush or loofah, working upwards in long sweeping strokes from your toes to your neck. Then wipe your body all over with a flannel or sponge and warm water. Now that you are nice and clean, you will not be sitting in your own dirt as you loll in the bath.

For deep-down cleanliness, you can give yourself a salt rub before you start. Add a little water – or milk, if your skin is very dry – to a cupful of sea-salt, and slather it over yourself from head to toe (except for your face and groin), rubbing it into your skin. Then sit down and the salt will dissolve into the water to give you a sea bath. If your skin is parched-dry, use a little oil instead of water to dampen the salt. 'Salt,' as Hungarian beauty specialist Countess Czaky was fond of telling her clients, 'preserves meat'.

You can do the same thing with magnesium sulphate or Epsom salts – very purifying. Or you can use **Oatmeal, Almond** meal, **Barley** meal or **Bran**, all cleansing and softening. Take a square of old cotton or linen sheet, tie the meal up in it with a firm knot, and put in your bath under the running tap. The milky liquid will soften your bath and your skin. Rub it all over yourself.

Milk itself is very soothing to the skin. Even a cupful of ordinary milk, or better still, instant dried non-fat milk added to the water will soften it a little; it is also an excellent medium for diluting and dispersing essential oils – add 5-6 drops of your favourite to a cupful.

A bath is a wonderful way to give yourself an aromatherapy treatment, but bear the following points in mind. The water should not be too hot, or the oils will evaporate too quickly. Be careful not to get the water in your eyes, as even the tiniest amount of oil could be irritat-

ing and damaging. Never forget that oils are extremely powerful concentrates of a plant, so do not use more than 5 drops in a bath. If you are using an oil for the first time, dilute it in milk or in another oil first; it might be one to which your skin is sensitive, and reacts with a blotchy rash or itching (I avoid **Lemon** for this reason). Do not use **Clary Sage** if you have been drinking alcohol; it could give you nightmares or have other strange effects.

N.B. Some essential oils should not be used during pregnancy: **Basil; Clove; Cinnamon; Hyssop; Juniper; Marjoram; Myrrh; Sage** and **Thyme. Fennel, Peppermint** and **Rosemary** should not be used during the first 4 months. Throughout pregnancy, use only half amounts of other oils – no more than 2 drops – in a bath.

If you have a treatment from a professional aromatherapist, she will also make up for you, if you ask, your own personal mix of the oils that suit your personality and any health problems you may have.

Among those she might use are: **Black Pepper** for aching muscles; **Clary Sage** as a pick-me-up – good for pre-menstrual tension, too; **Eucalyptus** if you have respiratory problems; **Geranium** for very dry or itchy skin, eczema, or PMS; **Jasmine** for when you wish to feel utterly luxurious – this costly oil is said to be an aphrodisiac; **Lavender** for dry skin, eczema, sprains, hot flushes, headaches, overwork, or – at bedtime – insomnia; **Neroli** for when you are feeling stressed and particularly fragile; **Orange** to pep you up; **Rosemary** to get you going in the morning – or in a quick pick-me-up bath before a busy social evening – good for aches and strained muscles, too. **Scotch Pine** is a bracing oil, excellent for colds and chesty problems, and useful if you perspire excessively; **Ylang-Ylang** is great for stress and tension, when you need cosseting.

Borax from any chemist is a cheap way to soften your bath-water if you live in a hard-water area. You can transform it into instant bath-salts, suggests Jeanne Rose, by adding some of your favourite essential oil. Put two cups of borax in a wide-mouthed jar, add 20-30 drops of oil and stir it all around with a wooden spoon. Repeat the next day, using another 20-30 drops. Close it up tightly after a few hours, and use 2-3 tablespoons in a bath.

If you are feeling chilled through, aching, pre-'flu-ish and generally out of sorts and low, try a **Ginger** bath; (see p.107 for how to prepare it).

In Ayurvedic medicine, milk is often used to extract herbs, particularly **Marshmallow** and **Comfrey**. Both are soothing and emollient herbs which are a good beauty treatment for dry and roughened skin, or skin dried out to the consistency of leather by weeks of baking Mediterranean sunshine. Use the ready-powdered roots, if you can get them, put a table-spoonful in a pan with 3 cups of milk, stir well, slowly heat, then simmer over a very low flame for 15 minutes. Strain into your bath.

You can use herbs for your bath in the form of an infused oil too; for instructions on how to make it, see p.144. **Chamomile, Lavender** or **Roses** are all good for dry, delicate or irritated skin; **Rosemary, Marigold** and **Thyme** for greasy skins; **Peppermint** for dull congested skin; **Geranium** leaves and flowers for all skin types. Stroke a palmful of the oil all over your body before you get into the bath.

Try mixing your infused oil with a treated Castor oil called Turkey Red, which – unlike most oils, which float on the surface – disperses in the water. Add 1 part of infused oil to 3 parts of Turkey Red, label it, put in a pretty bottle, and there is your luxurious bath oil.

Cider vinegar softens the skin, and helps preserve its acid mantle. But if you dislike the smell, use white wine vinegar instead. You can improve both the odour and the activity of either by half-filling a screw-top jar with aromatic herbs, filling it to the top with vinegar and letting them macerate for a week.

Try **Sage**, tonic and bracing; **Rosemary**, good for aching muscles, and very stimulating; **Thyme**, excellent for respiratory problems, rheumatism, and that run-down feeling; **Mint**, another stimulant; **Balm**, a real calmer; or **Marjoram**, a sedative, calming choice for bedtime.

Flower vinegars are lovely, too (see p.76 for how to make that stillroom classic, **Rose Vinegar**). Give the jar a shake from time to time, then strain out the herbs and decant into a pretty, clearly labelled, bottle.

A quicker way to prepare a herbal vinegar is as follows: put 1 cup of vinegar and 1 of water in a pan, bring to the boil and pour over 3 tablespoons of your chosen herb. Cover and let them steep for at least 12 hours, then strain. This is enough for 2 baths.

If you hanker for bubbles, buy a bottle of a good pH balanced shampoo, or a very mild baby shampoo; add a few drops of your favourite essential oil to it, and use it in the bath instead of on your hair.

For a herbal bath, you need a much stronger infusion than for drinking, because it will be so much more diluted. Take a good handful or two of the herb; add it to a panful of cold water, and bring it slowly to the boil. Turn the heat down very low, and simmer for at least 20 minutes. Strain and add to your bath. If you like, you can put the still-damp herbs in a square of linen or cotton, knot it firmly, and put it in your bath.

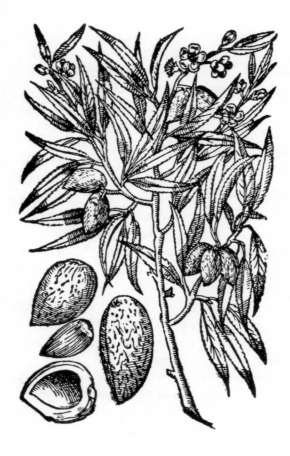

them, simply strain and tip into the bath. This is a wonderful softener and whitener for your skin.

Herb teabags can also be used up in your bath although you will need 4–6 to make a real impact. Leave them to infuse for at least 20 minutes. **Chamomile** is softening to the skin and calming for you; **Lime blossom** will help deep-cleanse your skin; **Fennel** is soothing and healing; **Peppermint** is stimulating, good for dull blotchy skin; **Nettles** are cleansing and nourishing to the skin.

If you are lucky enough to have your own herb-garden to pick from, you can prepare a cooling, refreshing **Lemon** bath on a hot day. Take a couple of handfuls of all the lemony herbs – **Lemon Verbena, Lemon Balm, Mint** and **Lemon Thyme** if you have it; put them in a pan with a twist of Lemon peel. Fill it up with cold water, bring to the boil, and simmer very gently covered for 20 minutes. Then strain into a luke-warm bath. Or infuse them all in a jarful of softening, nourishing **Avocado** or **Almond** oil for a real beauty treatment. Leave the jar tightly closed on a sunny window-sill, give it a shake from time to time, and strain out after 7–10 days.

In winter-time, you can make up a warming spicy bath. Put 10–12 **Cloves**, a piece of **Cinnamon** bark, and a twist of **Orange** peel in a pan; cover with cold water, and bring to the boil. Simmer covered for 20 minutes. Then strain and add to your bath. You can also use this mixture – adding a **Bay** leaf – to make up an infused oil.

If you go for a walk in a Pine forest, gather up a bagful of **Pine-cones**, take them home and dry them. Soak them overnight in a pan of cold water, when you are ready to use them;

Another way is to put a generous handful of herbs or flowers in a big thermos flask (keep an old one just for this); fill it up with boiling water, close, and let stand overnight or all day. Then strain and add to the bath.

Yet another way is to soak the herbs overnight in cold water; then bring them to the boil, simmer for just a minute, and leave to infuse for another 5–10 minutes. Strain and add to your bath.

One of the loveliest herbs to add to a bath, fortunately, grows in reckless profusion all over the countryside in May: **Elderflowers**. Take 4–5 of the big creamy heads when they are just flowering (after a day or two, a faint cat-like odour starts creeping into their perfume); soak them for at least 12 hours in a big bowl of cold water. When you are ready for bring the water with the cones in it just to the boil and simmer for no more than a minute. Leave to infuse for 10-15 minutes before straining and adding to your bath.

Finally, when you are bone-weary but sleepless at the end of a long day, make a strong infusion of **Hops** which will relax and soothe you. Put 2 tablespoons in a pint of water, simmer for 15 minutes covered, and then add to a bedtime bath.

HAIR

You cannot be beautiful, a well-known advertisement used to say, without beautiful hair. And you cannot have beautiful hair unless you are in good shape physically. This is a truth known to breeders: glossy coats are a sure sign that race-horses, dogs and cats are in tip-top condition. Show animals are often given special vitamin and mineral supplements to give them extra sheen for the big day.

Because it is the fastest-growing protein in our bodies, hair reflects our general state of health within days: when did you last see a sick friend with gloriously shiny hair? Alcoholic and gastronomic excesses, a bad bout of 'flu, a long period of stress or overwork – all of these will take the life and lustre out of your hair.

Switching to a healthier diet, with regular exercise, and a lower alcohol intake will bring almost immediate results in the shape of hair that seems suddenly thicker, shinier and easier to manage than the drab, thin stuff of a week or so ago.

Without good circulation in the scalp, the hair follicles will be starved of the nutrients supplied to them in the blood-stream. Many of the herbs traditionally used in hair-care – **Rosemary** is a prime example – stimulate local circulation. A gentle massage will help too. Curl and tense your fingers as though you were clutching a grapefruit in each hand. Apply your still-tensed fingers and the base of your palms to your scalp, and rock the scalp very gently for a minute or two. Then move to another area and start again, till your scalp has had a gentle all-over massage. Standing on your head is great, too, as is lying on a slant-board head-down. Just holding your head down in the traditional posture for a really good brushing has the same effect – a healthy rush of blood to the head.

Rosemary is a wonderful hair-tonic, and will cut down excess oiliness. Add a handful to 600ml/1 pint of cold water in a pan; bring to the boil and simmer for 15 minutes. Strain. Use this to swab the roots of your hair, all over your scalp; if possible leave on overnight before a morning shampoo. Add the rest of the infusion to the final rinse water.

Another way to give your hair the Rosemary treatment is by making up an infused oil; follow the technique described on p.144, and use as for Jojoba (see below).

Or you can make a non-greasy friction lotion by adding a teaspoon of essential oil of Rosemary to 100ml/3½floz of either vodka or gin. Shake very well. Use an hour or so before you shampoo.

Mexican women have always used **Jojoba** oil to make their hair thick and lustrous. This may be a purely cosmetic effect, since the oil smooths and coats the hair shafts. It is also believed by those who use it that it promotes hair growth, by the nourishment it supplies. If your hair looks dry and lacklustre, try the

Jojoba oil treatment. Heat up a couple of table-spoons of Jojoba oil – stand the bottle in a basin of very hot water for a few minutes. Section your hair, apply it to the roots all over your scalp, then comb it right through the rest of your hair. Wrap a warm towel round your head, and leave on for 30 minutes. Then use a very mild shampoo, rinsing your hair thoroughly. Jojoba oil is quite expensive, and it can be diluted with **Sweet Almond** oil, which is itself a good conditioning treatment for the hair.

An oil treatment does not sound like a very good way to get rid of dandruff, or treat greasy hair. But in fact research has established Jojoba's ability to inhibit excess activity of the sebaceous glands.

Eastern women use **Ginger** root and **Sesame** oil for a conditioning treatment that counters dandruff and falling hair. Grate a piece of the fresh root, squeeze out the juice into an equal quantity of Sesame oil. Section the hair bit by bit, apply the oil all over the scalp. Wrap a warm towel round your head and leave on as long as possible before shampooing out. Sesame seeds are wonderful nourishment for the hair, high in minerals such as iron and zinc, and antioxidant vitamin E – eat plenty of them.

Macrobiotic teacher Michio Kushi suggests a course of Sesame seed tea to help restore colour to dark hair. Add a cupful of water to 2-3 teaspoons of Sesame seeds and bring to the boil; simmer for 15-20 minutes. Drink 2-3 cups a day for 2-3 weeks. The rich nutrients in Sesame seeds will also benefit your vision. You can enhance the Sesame treatment by applying it straight to your hair. Crush 2 tea-spoons of the seeds and simmer them in a cup-ful of water for 15-20 minutes; strain and use as a final rinse after shampoo. Leave on the hair as long as possible before rinsing off.

Any patch of waste land will supply the raw materials for one of the oldest and most highly-respected treatments for hair problems – **Nettles**. In addition to their cleansing, tonic and astringent action, Nettles are rich in the minerals which hair needs for healthy growth; these include iron, sulphur and silicon, as well as beta-carotene, vitamin C and chlorophyll. One of the simplest ways to give your hair this nutritious treat – from the inside as well as the outside – is to gather a big panful of very young Nettle-tops, put them with a table-spoonful of water in a pan, to cook like spinach. Once cooked, strain off the juice, eat the Nettles as a vegetable with plenty of butter and a little Nutmeg; save the juice to cool and use as hair-friction, rubbing it well into the scalp. Repeat the friction every other night for 2-3 weeks, and your hair will be healthy, soft and glossy.

A hair tonic that will keep longer is made by steeping the carefully washed, whole young Nettle plant – roots and all – in 2 parts of water to 1 of Cider vinegar to cover. Bring to the boil and simmer for 30 minutes; then strain and add one third part of eau de cologne. The roots are also used on their own, macerated overnight in a panful of cold water. In the morning, bring to boiling point, simmer for 5 minutes, and strain. Use for your morning shampoo.

As a daily scalp friction, make up a Nettle root tincture, using a handful of the finely chopped roots in enough alcohol to cover completely; leave to macerate for a fortnight.

Burdock, the great mineral-rich cleanser, is another fine hedgerow remedy for frail, falling hair. The fresh root should be used: put a good handful, carefully cleaned, in a litre/1¾ pints of water. Simmer for about 20 minutes, and use as a scalp friction; then use a very mild shampoo. The rest of the decoction can be the final rinse, and leave your hair to dry naturally if possible.

Combine the fresh roots of Burdock and Nettle in this French remedy for thinning hair: 100g/4oz of Burdock root, 50g/2oz of Nettle root chopped up very small and macerated in 500ml/¾ pint of rum for 8-10 days and carefully strained. Friction daily with this.

Both Burdock and Nettle will help your hair – and you – from the inside too; try a week's course of 2-3 cups a day of an infusion of either. Infuse a handful of Nettle leaves for 10 minutes in a litre/1¾ pints of water, or 1tsp of Burdock root simmered for 10 minutes in a cupful of water.

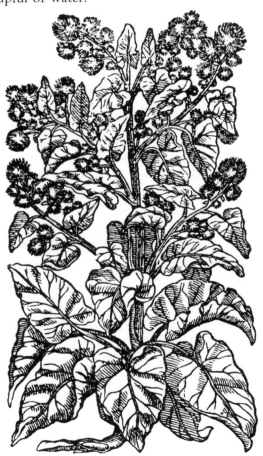

Dr Valnet suggests combining Burdock root with **Wild Thyme**, another great hair tonic. Simmer a handful of each in a litre/1¾ pints of water for 15 minutes, and use as a scalp friction twice a week.

You need plenty of sulphur in your diet for thick, healthy hair; sulphur binds amino acids in the hair shaft, and a deficiency may be giving your hair a dead or brittle look.

You may feel, though, that you would rather have brittle hair than try this old country cure – a raw **Onion** (Onions are *very* rich in sulphur) rubbed over the roots of your hair before you shampoo it! For a more refined version of the Onion cure, peel and slice a nice fat Onion; put it in a jar and cover it with gin or vodka. Leave it for a day or two, then start swabbing your hair roots with the mix (leave the Onion in). If even the Onion tincture offends your nose, just eat plenty of Onions. Eat lots of **Watercress, Cabbage, Broccoli** and **Radish** too – all sulphur-rich foods.

Another sulphur-rich plant with a long reputation in hair-care is the bright **Nasturtium**: 100g/4oz of the plant contains up to 170mg of sulphur. It is highly regarded by French herbalists, who recommend it for every kind of hair problem, from excess greasiness to thinning and weakening of the hair, or premature baldness following serious illness or treatment with certain drugs.

You can make a simple decoction of the flowers, leaves and stems – a handful simmered for 15 minutes, then strained and used as a friction and final rinse. Or you can make this more elaborate friction lotion – which will keep for months – and use it regularly. Take 100g/4oz each of fresh flowers and seeds of Nasturtium; and fresh Nettles; finely chop and macerate in 500ml/¾ pint of vodka for a fortnight; press out, strain and bottle. Add a couple of drops of your favourite essential oil – perhaps **Rosemary** or **Geranium** – to give it a nice smell.

Watercress is a close relation of Nasturtium, and equally well endowed with sulphur and other vital minerals. It was warmly recommended by the School of Salerno as a hair-conditioner.

The School of Salerno also recommended yolk of egg, yet another good source of sulphur, which presumably is why it is so often suggested as a hair-conditioner. Ever since I ended up with a head full of scrambled eggs, after rinsing with much too hot water, I have not been keen on this one, personally. If you're less faint-hearted, there are some excellent versions of the egg-treatment.

WHOLE EGG CONDITIONER FOR DULL, BRITTLE HAIR

Beat 2 eggs until fluffy. Work them carefully into clean hair. Leave this on for ½ hour or more. Rinse it out with warm water, followed by a shampoo, a vinegar rinse, and more warm water to leave hair healthy and shining.

Mother Nature's Beauty Cupboard
(Donna Lawson, 1973)

Silicon is just as vital to the hair as to the skin: and much of the body's silicon is concentrated in the hair. For silicon-rich foods, see p. 92.

Many commercial shampoos are alkaline, and however squeaky-clean they may leave your hair, they also strip off the acid mantle of the scalp, and the protective film of sebum on the hair-shafts; this leaves the scalp dry and your hair lifeless. You can restore the balance by adding a tablespoonful of **Cider** vinegar to the final rinse water which will leave your hair soft and glossy, as well as clean.

Use Cider vinegar as the basis of an effective friction rub, using **Rosemary** for any colour hair, including grey, **Sage** for dark hair, **Chamomile** for fair hair. Take a handful of the fresh herb, or 25g/1oz of the dried; put in a pan with 500ml/¾ pint of water and bring to the boil. Simmer for 10 minutes. Strain and mix with an equal quantity of Cider vinegar. Cool before bottling and labelling carefully.

I remember being very jealous of my blonde sister Hilda, when we were little girls submitting to the weekly shampoo. Her hair was carefully rinsed afterwards with a jugful of a fragrant golden liquid, which I watched being made from the papery heads of **Chamomile** – a very old European beauty secret. My straight brown hair got an ordinary shampoo. But just one Chamomile teabag will not do much for blondes: you need 2 heaped tbsp of the dried herb, and it should be simmered in 600ml of water for 20 minutes before straining for use. Swab it all over your hair before you shampoo, combing it right through. Then use the rest for the final rinse, after shampooing. Keep pouring the infusion over and over, collecting it in a basin and pouring it again. Blot your hair dry, and dry naturally.

Marigold flowers, **Cowslips** and the lovely bright yellow flowers of **Great Mullein** have all traditionally been used to highlight fair hair, sometimes combined with Chamomile. Beauty secrets for brunettes also exist.

In an article in *The Herbalist*, Dorothy Crisp suggests infusing 2tbsp each of Red Sage and Rosemary in 600ml/1 pint of water. 'If used regularly,' she says, this 'will gradually darken the hair as well as giving an extremely attractive perfume.'

If you have a **Walnut** tree growing in your garden, you can make up this Italian prescription for healthy, glossy dark hair. Take a handful of the leaves and 3-4 of the green husks. Put them in a pan with a 1½ litres/2½ pints of water, bring to the boil and simmer for 20 minutes. Strain and use as the final rinse after shampooing. Let your hair dry naturally, so that the rinse remains in contact with it as long as possible. The leaves are said to contain traces of iodine, which might explain why they make hair look so good; without iodine, the thyroid gland – which ensures the circulation in the scalp – will be underactive. A final rinse with a strong infusion of **Sage** is also said to help darken hair – it will certainly have a conditioning effect. And one French remedy for that distressing condition *alopecia*, is regular friction rubs with a lotion composed of equal parts of rum and tincture of Sage (a herbalist will supply this, or you can make your own – (see p.143).

The Japanese believe that eating lots of **Seaweed** will help keep their hair strong, dark, thick and glossy. Seaweeds are rich in iodine, iron and sulphur – all minerals that healthy hair needs.

Lucky redheads can condition their hair while they dye it anything from pale marmalade to deep amber, with the help of **Henna**. Arab women have used Henna for centuries, not only to care for and colour their hair, but also as medicine, according to Juliette de Baïracli Levy. The ground-up dried root, bark, berries and small greyish-green leaves of this oriental shrub are made up into a cooling clay to use in fevers, or to cleanse the body of impurities. She reminds us that Henna is quite astringent, so a bland oil should be rubbed into the hair after a treatment, if it seems too dry. If on the other hand your hair is inclined to be greasy,

this is another plus for Henna. You can buy pure Henna from herbal suppliers and the Body Shop.

Take a **Lemon**, wash it carefully and slice it; remove the pips, and reduce it – in a blender or food processor – to a smooth pulp. Filter it through muslin, and mix with equal parts of **Cider** vinegar. After washing and rinsing your hair, blot it dry with a towel, and then give your scalp a light but thorough friction with the Lemon-vinegar mixture. Leave it on for 5-10 minutes, then rinse off. This will leave your hair gloriously clean, grease-free and shining, and your scalp will feel extra-clean and fresh.

Did you ever wonder where the charming little **Maidenhair** fern – otherwise known as Hair of Venus – got its name? It may be because it has a long history of country use as a remedy for both dandruff and falling hair. Italians make a decoction of 15g of the fresh herb in 150ml/¼ pint of water, simmered for 10 minutes, and used as a friction 3 times a week.

AROMATIC VINEGARS
Steep 1oz fresh Rosemary and 1oz fresh Mint, preferably bergamot Mint, in enough white vinegar to cover for 2-3 weeks. Strain. This is an excellent vinegar to use after your shampoo to rid yourself of dandruff.

Herbs and Things
(Jeanne Rose, 1972)

Tea Tree oil has remarkable solvent properties which can be particularly helpful if you have a scaly, itchy scalp. This is often due to a build-up of dead cells, and to clogged hair follicles. When you add Tea Tree to your shampoo, inpacted sebum or cellular debris is washed away with the rinsing water. It is an excellent dandruff treatment, for the same reason. There are Tea Tree oil shampoos on the market; or you can add a few drops of the oil to an ordinary shampoo. Its clean, antiseptic action will help clear any local infections too.

At one time or another most mothers have opened one of those dreaded letters from their children's school warning of a current plague of nits, those nasty little creatures which hop so quickly from one child to another, no matter how clean and shiny the hair. I never wanted to cover my daughters' heads with the strongly chemical and vile-smelling anti-nit shampoo recommended on these occasions. I was therefore delighted when a suggestion in Maggie Tisserand's *Aromatherapy for Women* not only worked like a charm, but left their hair particularly glossy and healthy-looking. This is what she suggests: To 75ml/2½floz of oil (use a bland Almond or Sunflower oil) add the following essential oils: 25 drops each of **Rosemary** and **Lavender**, 12 drops of **Eucalyptus**; 13 drops of **Geranium**. Section the hair carefully, applying the oil mixture to the roots all over the head; then carefully comb the oil all through the hair. Pile it on top of the head, then wrap clingfilm tightly around it. Leave on for a couple of hours. Then shampoo and use a fine-toothed comb to comb out the now-dead nits. Repeat after 2 weeks.

Tea Tree oil is another effective treatment for nits. Use a Tea Tree oil shampoo boosted with 10-12 drops of the pure oil – or add 15-20 drops to an ordinary shampoo. Leave the shampoo on for 10 minutes, then rinse out, and repeat a week later.

Aromatherapy is not just a luxurious way to improve the health and look of your hair; it is also simplicity itself. To make up a useful friction for your scalp, add 10 drops of essential oil to a little bottle of vodka – label the bottle! – and use for a regular scalp treatment. **West Indian Bay** is useful for all hair problems; **Bergamot** or **Geranium** are good for greasy hair; **Rosemary** or **Lavender** for dry hair.

EYES

The incredibly tough yet extraordinarily delicate human eye is built to take a lot of punishment. Nature has devised an intriguing array of protective devices for its safety. It is sunk in a bony socket to guard it from blows, falls or other accidents. The eyebrows mop up any sweat that might otherwise trickle down into the eyes. The eyelids blink open and shut to keep out dust, dirt and other hostile flying objects; and if anything gets through, they will blink even faster to help clear it almost before you know there is anything wrong. Eyelashes are extra protection, trapping dust particles or droplets of liquid – in a blizzard, they will soon be thick and white with snow. The eyeball itself is encased in a very tough membrane called the cornea, which can survive – and recover quite rapidly from – even severe injuries. Finally, the eyes are constantly bathed in a liquid secreted by the tear ducts which contains a germicidal compound.

Nature has done her best for the eyes, so what can we ourselves do to keep them clear, bright and sparkling? A great deal, fortunately.

We can make sure that we eat plenty of the foods particularly important to their health and well-being (see What Is Healthy Eating, p.22). Vitamin A is especially important; severe deficiency will eventually lead to blindness, and if your night vision is poor, you are already short of it. Your diet should also supply high levels of antioxidants, essential fatty acids, zinc and protein.

He who suffers in his stomach or his intestines because he has poor digestion, his eyes will become enfeebled.
Manuel de la Medecine
de Ste. Hildegarde
(Herttzka (ed.), 1988)

Stress is always reflected in your eyes, which are directly connected to the brain (see The Nervous System, which has suggestions to help you cope with stress).

Alcohol, smoking, all forms of pollution and a number of prescription drugs, can have an adverse effect on eyes in a number of ways. They drain the body of vital nutrients, and generate free radicals, which have been pinpointed as a major cause of cataracts and other damage to the eyes.

Eyes depend on good circulation to keep them supplied with the nutrients they need; and to remove wastes which might irritate or damage them. So exercise will benefit them too; and if you practise yoga, those head- and shoulder-stands will do wonders for them.

There are a number of herbs which will help you refresh your eyes; soothe them when they are red, sore or irritated; tone the tiny muscles that keep them functioning; help them overcome infections; and stimulate local microcirculation to keep the sparkle in them.

N.B. For all their built-in protective devices, eyes are very susceptible to infection, particularly when you are under stress. Anything that touches them – hands, eyebaths, linen or cotton for compresses – should be scrupulously clean. Herbal infusions for use in or on the eyes should be made with spring or distilled water, extra-carefully strained through coffee filter-paper, and used as soon as possible. Compresses *on* the eyes can be used at any time, but washes and drops *in* the eyes should be used only for severe irritation, soreness, redness and infection.

Carrots are a Super Food for the eyes; pilots during World War II were officially encouraged to eat plenty of them, and huntsmen in Switzerland drink a twice-daily glass of Carrot juice to keep their vision sharp during the hunting season. Eat plenty of **Bilberries** too (see p.45).

Sesame seeds are traditionally eaten by Oriental women to help overcome eye problems. They are rich in protein, zinc and vitamin E, all vital to eye health.

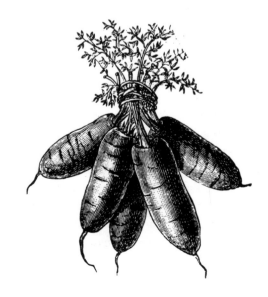

Eyebright has for centuries enjoyed a firm reputation as a remedy in eye problems, as its popular names suggest: *brise-lunettes* – break-spectacles in French, *augentrost* or consolation of the eyes, in German. A particular tannin it contains may be responsible for its power to soothe and counter inflammation. It may also act on the local circulation, and is traditionally recommended for the memory too. Herbalists prescribe it for conjunctivitis, watering or inflamed eyes and weakness of the sight.

The juice or distilled water of Eyebright, taken inwardly in white wine or broth, or dipped into the eyes, for divers days together, helps all infirmities of the eyes that cause dimness of sight. Some make conserve of the flowers to the same effect. Being used any of these ways, it also helps a weak brain, or memory.

The Complete Herbal
(Nicholas Culpeper)

Eyebright is taken internally as well as being used on the eyes themselves: Put 1 tsp of the flowering stems in a cupful of water, boil for 1 minute and leave to infuse for 5 minutes. Drink a cupful 3 times a day between meals for 1 week. For external use, use 1 tsp of the dried herb to 500ml/¾ pint of water, boil for 1 minute, then leave to infuse for 30 minutes. Soak a linen or cotton compress in the carefully strained infusion when it has cooled a little; cover the eyes and forehead, then lie down and think tranquil thoughts for 15 minutes. Repeat 2-3 times a day. Alternatively, add 30 drops of the tincture of Eyebright to ½ cupful of cold purified water and use this in a compress.

The petals of red **Roses** are another traditional favourite for eye-care, especially for inflamed or irritated eyelids. Make a cooling and soothing compress of the petals to refresh tired eyes. Or make a lotion by infusing 2-3 pinches of the petals in a glassful of boiling water for 10 minutes; cool, strain and use in a cold compress. In the form of distilled water, Roses are often combined with Eyebright in a lotion for the eyes. Add 30 drops of the tincture to a wineglassful of Rose water; use to bathe the eyes, or as a cold compress (label it carefully, and keep it in the fridge).

The beautiful blue **Cornflower** and the healing **Plantain** are two other herbs prescribed by herbalists to treat conjunctivitis and other eye problems. They are combined with Eyebright in this French prescription: take 5oz of Eyebright and 25g/1oz each of Cornflowers and Plantain leaves; pour 100ml/3½floz of boiling water over a soup-spoonful of this mixture and leave to infuse for 30 minutes, then strain and cool. Use in eyebaths or cold compresses.

Infusions of **Chamomile** and **Marigold** used in a cold compress are calming and soothing to troubled eyes. **Witch-Hazel** – especially ice-cold straight from the fridge – is another wonderful refresher for tired, bleary eyes; soak pads of cotton wool and put them over closed eyes while you put your feet up for 10 minutes. Witch-Hazel is often combined with Rose water in eyebaths or compresses.

Fennel has an age-old reputation in the maintenance of eye health, whether you eat the root and feathery tops as a vegetable, or first thing in the morning drink a tea made from the seeds. Try an infusion of the seeds: 1tbsp of the crushed seeds simmered for 5 minutes in 600ml/1pint of water, strained and cooled, used as a compress several times a day for conjunctivitis or sore red eyes.

---

*Whoever eats daily of Fennel or its seeds
fasting will find they dispel much
unhealthy mucus or putrefaction in himself
and banish the evil odour of his breath and
enable his eyes to see well again, restoring
good warmth and strength.*

(St Hildegarde of Bingen)

In his lovely book *Natural Folk Remedies*, US health writer Lelord Kordel lists a number of remedies collected around the world for eye problems. An English remedy is 3 tbsp of **Honey** diluted in 2 cups of boiling water, stirred until dissolved, then cooled and used in an eyebath. Hollywood actors, like so many others, discovered the benefits of the **Cabbage**; eyes strained by the day-long glare of studio lighting were given poultices of Cabbage leaves softened – but not cooked – in boiling water.

Two kitchen remedies for tired eyes: a compress made of very finely grated raw **Potato** in a piece of sterile gauze can be laid gently over the eyes – or even the Potato slices themselves; and to cool down inflamed and burning eyes, use a compress of finely grated **Cucumber**.

Mouth, Teeth and Gums

It is something of a shock to realize that half the great beauties of history probably had rotten teeth. Dentistry is one of the great achievements of our time, and we should be thankful for it. With our modern diet, we need it: shrinking, diseased gums, teeth decaying and becoming 'unfastened' – as they used to say in the old herbals – are still sadly common, even among those who visit their dentist regularly.

The gums, the inside of the mouth and the tongue are the upper and visible end of our lengthy digestive tracts; any trouble brewing in the digestive system is almost immediately reflected in the condition of the mouth. Till quite recently, every GP used to ask patients to put out their tongue – as traditional Chinese doctors still do – because it is such a good indication of the state of health of the digestive tract. Vitamin B deficiencies show up here almost instantly; if you are short of vitamin C, your gums will bleed easily – sailors afflicted with scurvy often lost all their teeth. Eat plenty of wholegrains for B-complex and minerals; if possible eat organically grown fruit and vegetables, free from pesticides. Otherwise wash the skins thoroughly; they are rich in the silicon that is indispensable for sound strong teeth (see Skin, p.73).

Some people start life with strong, white, healthy teeth and never have any trouble with them, whatever their diet. Others have dim, lacklustre teeth and endless cavities. It is partly the luck of the draw, but if you were not born with wonderful teeth, there is plenty you can do to strengthen them, and to ensure that firm healthy gums keep them 'fastened' for the term of your natural life.

It is common sense to have regular checkups with your dentist, and to make sure that your teeth and gums are well nourished from the inside too.

There are herbs that will help keep your teeth strong, your gums firm and full, your tongue tingly-clean, and your breath as fresh as a rose. Since the mucous membrane of the mouth and gums is highly absorbent, so both nutrients and compounds with a specific pharmacological action are rapidly absorbed into the bloodstream from herbs held in the mouth in the form of a mouthwash, or applied directly to the gums.

Aloe Vera can make an impressive contribution to dental health and hygiene. It speeds healing of damaged tissue, counters irritation and inflammation, and has a slight local numbing effect, useful after dental surgery or for mouth or gum ulcers. Apply a little of it directly to the gums. It fights infection too; tests cited in Diane Gage's book *Aloe Vera* have shown it to be effective against 5 different strains of 1 micro-organism which causes tooth decay.

In the 1930s dentists around the world began enthusiastically using **Tea Tree** oil from Australia; it had been hailed in the scientific press as 'non-toxic, non-irritating, and 11 to 13 times stronger than carbolic as a germicide'. Tea Tree, sadly, has been largely forgotten by dentists as an oral antiseptic and in oral hygiene. But millions of people are discovering how clean, fresh and healthy Tea Tree can help keep their mouth and gums.

Tea tree is lethal to an extraordinarily wide range of infective micro-organisms, including most of those responsible for tooth decay and gum disease. If you have shrinking gums with pockets around the teeth that easily become infected, a daily rinse with Tea Tree, as well as regular check-ups with a dentist, should take care of the problem. Tea Tree can be dabbed straight on to problem gums with a cotton wool bud, or used as a mouthwash; add 3-4 drops of Tea Tree to a coffee-cup of water and gently swill around the mouth.

Propolis is a sticky, resinous substance gathered by industrious bees from the leaf-buds and barks of certain trees, and plastered all over hives the way builders use cement. The astonishing antibiotic properties of this substance have been shown in clinical studies to be spectacularly effective against infections of the throat and the mouth. Among the constituents of Propolis are a number of flavonoids, which may contribute to its anti-inflammatory action, and its stimulating effect on local circulation. It also contains traces of a number of minerals vital to healthy teeth, bone and connective tissue, including silicon and iron. Thus Propolis is not only a powerful local antiseptic that soothes, has a mild local anaesthetic effect and speeds healing, but is also a source of important nutrients for the whole mouth area. As such, it figures in many different products.

You can use Propolis as a tincture; dab it straight on to mouth ulcers – much the most effective treatment I know for the pain and discomfort they cause; or use a cotton wool bud to treat awkward corners of the gums; or sprinkle a few drops on a toothbrush to work all the way round teeth and gums. Try adding a teaspoonful to half a glass of water, and use as a mouthwash or gargle. You can also chew Propolis lozenges, and there are Propolis toothpastes on the market.

Sesame and **Sunflower** seeds are loaded with minerals badly needed for strong teeth and healthy gums. Chew them slowly.

Modern herbalists use **Echinacea** to counter infection and boost your immune response. Use ½ tsp of the tincture in half-a-glass of water, as a mouthwash; this leaves your entire mouth feeling fresh, and will help firm and tone gums.

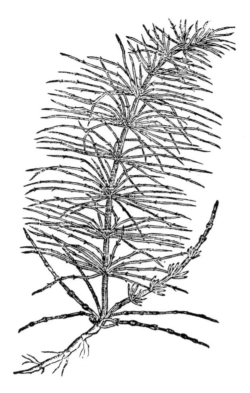

No other herb is richer in silicon than **Horsetail**; when you gargle with an infusion of it, you are giving teeth, bones and gums a useful dose. Because of the role silicon plays in connective tissue, Horsetail is also healing for sores and wounds. Lesley Tierra gives a wonderful formula for a home-made tooth-powder featuring Horsetail. Combine equal parts of powdered **Myrrh, Cinnamon, Bayberry bark, Horsetail** and **Echinacea**. Then add ½ parts of powdered **Prickly Ash, Cayenne** and baking soda. Myrrh is an age-old remedy for wounds, highly valued in Ancient Greece for its antiseptic and healing powers. Astringent Bayberry bark will firm and tone gums. Settlers in North America christened Prickly Ash the 'Toothache tree' once they had learned its antiseptic and healing powers from the native Indians. Cayenne will give a powerful jolt to the local circulation. 'I have one friend,' relates Lesley, 'who prevented gum surgery by just brushing her teeth daily with Cayenne powder.'

Tincture of **Myrrh** is a great herbal standby for any infections of the mouth or gums, which it can clean up and heal with remarkable speed. It has a firming and stimulating effect on gums, too, although it has a very bitter taste; add 3-4 drops to half-a-glass of water to rinse around your mouth.

Refer to First Aid, p.145, for the use of Cloves for toothache and in clearing up gum infections.

Nobody needs an excuse to enjoy **Strawberries** in the summer, but in case you do, tell yourself that they are amazingly good for you, and will give you white, tartar-free teeth – as long as you eat enough of them.

Bilberries are another fruit that can do wonders for dental hygiene. Their astringency and antiseptic powers make them effective for mouth ulcers or sores and infections in the gums; take a mouthful of them and chew them very, very slowly. You can spit them out afterwards if you want to.

All the berries are rich sources of minerals, vitamin C and beta-carotene, as well as flavonoids and other compounds with a marked antiseptic action. Eat them slowly, so that some of their nutrients are absorbed by the mucous membrane to fortify gums and teeth. **Blackcurrants** and **Cherries** are also good for the mouth; in one study, a compound in black Cherries was shown to help block plaque formation.

Blackberry leaves were an old country stand-in for ordinary tea, in the days when it was still a high-priced luxury. Those drinking it may have noticed how much healthier their teeth and gums were looking; Blackberry leaves have always been famous for their tonic, antiseptic and regenerative action on the mucous membranes of the mouth. Chew them while they're green and fresh (like the Bilberries, you can spit them out afterwards).

Once a week – but not more often – brush your teeth with freshly-pressed **Lemon** juice.

It is very lowering to the spirits to be told you have bad breath. Maybe it is a dental problem? Or something amiss down in the digestive tract? Try any of the following. Brush your teeth very thoroughly, then put a couple of drops of **Tea Tree** oil or tincture of **Propolis** on your toothbrush for a final rinse. Chew **Mint** leaves; fresh **Parsley**; fresh **Tarragon; Fennel** seeds; **Coffee** beans; **Cardamom** pods or **Cumin** seeds; or add a drop of the essential oil of **Peppermint** to a tablespoon of vodka or milk, and swish it round your mouth for a couple of minutes. Crush a few **Cloves** and simmer them in a cupful of boiling water for 5 minutes, cool and use as a mouthwash. You can also make up a strong infusion of **Lavender, Rosemary** or **Sage**, to use as a mouthwash. The delightful thing about any of these is that not only will they sweeten your breath, they are also a grand tonic for your teeth and gums; if it *is* a dental problem that is responsible for your less-than-fresh breath, they will get to work on that, too.

Sage is particularly tonic and stimulating to the gums and mucous membrane. Women used to rub fresh Sage leaves on their teeth to make them whiter and improve their gums; if you have a healthy Sage plant in your garden or on your window-sill, follow their example. You can also make your own Sage toothpowder as follows. Pick a couple of handfuls of the leaves, wash them, crush them in a pes-

tle and mortar and put them in a small oven-proof dish with a tablespoonful of sea salt. Mix together and bake in a moderate oven till the leaves are crisp and dry, then grind to powder in a coffee mill and use daily. You can make **Horsetail** toothpowder the same way, or you can mix them. An infusion of **Sage** – 4–5 leaves to a cupful of boiling water, infused covered for 5 minutes – makes an excellent antiseptic mouthwash with a cool fresh taste. Add just a pinch of **Cayenne** to reinforce its action.

Roses can be powerful medicine; it is generally agreed among herbalists that the deep red ones are more potent than the paler colours or white. If you have red Roses in your garden, gather up some of the petals when they are full blown, put them in a basin, and pour boiling water over them. If the water slowly turns a beautiful deep rose colour, you can use them for a particularly effective mouthwash, cleansing and strengthening to the gums and mucous membrane. Better still, make a vinegar extract. Put 60g/2½oz of the petals in 750ml/1¼ pints of a good red wine vinegar, so that they are completely covered; close the jar, and leave to macerate for a week. Give them a shake from time to time. Strain, decant the wonderful deep red liquid into an attractive bottle, label clearly, and keep it in your bathroom. Every now and then put a tablespoon or so in a little glass of warm water, and have a gargle.

Tonic and purifying **Burdock** is destructive to a number of the micro-organisms responsible for mouth and gum infections. Make a decoction with 1 teaspoon of the root simmered in a cupful of water for 15 minutes. Use a mouthwash, holding it in your mouth for minutes at a time while you read a good book; spit this out then drink the rest as a tea.

Agrimony contains traces of silicon as well as iron and some B vitamins; it is tonic, healing, bracing for the gums. Make an infusion by pouring a cupful of boiling water over 1½tsp of the dried herb, and leaving to infuse for 10–15 minutes.

If you are feeling brave, try chewing on a piece of **Horseradish** root. Rich in minerals, including cleansing sulphur, and high in vitamin C, it is regarded a great general stimulant – but not for the faint-hearted. . . .

A Mediterranean remedy for bleeding and infected gums is as follows. Simmer a good pinch of **Olive** leaves covered in 200ml/⅓ pint of water for about 20 minuts. Cool, strain, and use as a mouthwash.

Houseleek leaves are also astringent and healing; chew a leaf and keep it in your mouth for a moment or so.

Skin

The best skin food ever invented is just that: good food. Eat well, and you will look well.

There are wonder Foods, however, which do a particularly good job of nourishing your skin from the inside. Eat plenty of the bright red, yellow, orange and green fruits and vegetables: **Apricots; Oranges; Peppers; Carrots; Strawberries;** and **Broccoli**. They are rich in carotenoid pigments, which your body converts to vitamin A – vital for healthy skin – and many other nutrients (some still unidentified).

Include the blood-cleansing, blood-building mineral-rich greens such as **Dandelion, Nettles, bitter Chicory, Watercress, Chickweeds** in your diet. They are high in blood-enriching chlorophyll, too.

Sunflower, Pumpkin and **Sesame** seeds are rich in zinc and other minerals vital to the health, repair and maintenance of a beautiful skin. And make sure your diet supplies the essential fatty acids, from oily fish like mackerel, sardines and salmon, and from extra virgin **Olive** oil.

One mineral that is very important to the skin is silicon. Little research has yet been done into this major mineral, the importance of which is demonstrated by the amounts of it found in our bodies – nearly half as much as zinc. Much of this silicon is found in healthy connective tissue, on which the soft suppleness of the skin depends.

For more about silicon and which foods or herbs supply it, see The Circulatory System, p.92. For suggestions on diet, or help with specific skin problems such as acne, see the chapter on The Skin, in Part 3 'Remedies', p.85.

Watercress. . . . The leaves bruised, or the juice, is good to be applied to the face or other parts troubled with freckles, pimples, spots or the like, at night, and washed away in the morning. . . . Watercress pottage is a good remedy to cleanse the blood in the spring . . . and consume the gross humours winter hath left behind: those that would live in health may use it if they please, if they will not I cannot help it. If any fancy not pottage, they may eat the herb as a salad.

The Complete Herbal
(Nicholas Culpeper)

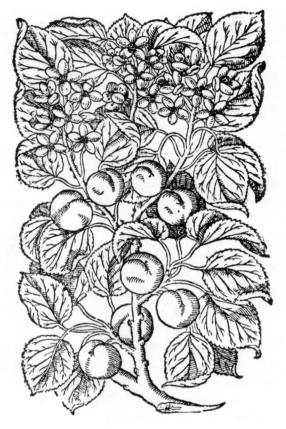

Some of the best skin-foods work well from
the outside; being rapidly absorbed by the
skin, the nutrients go straight to their target.
This is why in cosmetic science the big-name
beauty houses are rushing out skin-care products containing antioxidants, to counteract
the free-radical activity which produces ageing
and wrinkled skin. Fruits and vegetables
applied to the skin also have a number of tonic,
stimulating, soothing or vitalizing effects
locally.

The new buzzword in skin-care is AHAs, or
alpha hydroxy-acids; first formulated in the
1970s by cosmetic chemists, they are based on
acids found in Citrus fruits, Grapes, and Passion fruit, among others, as well as lactic acid
(found in whey). The AHAs work their magic
by correcting skin pH to its optimum level,
allowing it to slough off the top layer of dead
skin cells. In young skins, these dead cells are
shed routinely; but in ageing skin, they can
accumulate to give it a dull and lifeless look,
and accentuate tiny wrinkles. The discovery
provides a rationale for the centuries-old use of
Orange or Lemon juice directly on the skin –
and no doubt of other fruits long popular as
beauty aids. The effectiveness of AHA-based
creams now on the market emphasizes once
more the vital importance of the skin's acid
mantle.

Carrot juice helps keep skin fresh and supple,
and clears imperfections; it supplies plenty of
beta-carotene and vitamin C.

Tomatoes firm, tone and freshen skin; they
also help eliminate blackheads. **Lettuce** juice
added to whipped egg-white is also excellent
for blackheads.

Cucumber juice soothes and softens skin;
use it after going out in biting winds, or strong
sunshine. It also keeps the skin clear. Grate the
Cucumber into a little yoghurt or cream; this
will cool and calm inflamed or blotchy skin.

Avocados supply nourishing and easily

absorbed oils especially welcome to a dry skin; they are rich in antioxidants A and E, with a little vitamin C. Israaeli research has shown that substances in Avocado flesh can trigger the production of more embryonal collagen, the soluble kind that gives babies their soft skin. The oil – which you can use on its own – penetrates through the dermis and epidermis to deliver its wealth of nutrients to first base. Next time you eat an Avocado, save some of the flesh. Smooth it over your face and let it firm for 10-15 minutes; then rinse it off with warm water. Or simply run the creamy inside of the skin over your face.

On your Mediterranean holiday, when the local market is full of soft ripe **Apricots**, save one and rub the soft juicy flesh over your face. This is a wonderful tonic for your skin; Apricots are also rich in antioxidant beta-carotene, which you need to protect your skin from the sun.

Apple juice is a year-round tonic, which helps firm the skin of face and neck. Swab it on generously with cotton wool; leave it for a few minutes, then rinse off.

Lemon juice is another cosmetic fruit with an age-old reputation in skin-care. It is especially good for greasy skin; swab it on after your bedtime skin-cleansing and let it dry on the skin overnight. Lemon juice boosts the micro-circulation of the skin, lightens its colour, and helps remove blackheads and other blemishes. Its high antioxidant content makes Lemon juice an excellent treatment for wrinkles; Danièle Ryman suggests diluting it with distilled or mineral water and massaging it gently into wrinkles, especially round the mouth and eyes.

For thousands of years, the **Rose** has been a metaphor for feminine beauty, prized for its fragrance as much as for its glowing colours. As recently as this century, chemists still sup-plied Rose Honey, Rose Syrup, Confection of Roses, Rose Water Ointment, and a Rose Lotion made with Almonds, beeswax, spermaceti and oils of Bergamot and Lavender, among other things. Chemists still sell distilled Rose Water, one of the cheapest mild and soothing astringents available, and an ingredient in many do-it-yourself herbal cosmetics.

Generations of women have distilled their own **Elderflower** water, stimulating, mildly astringent, and – they believed – whitening to the skin.

Three herbs turn up over and over again in 'natural' skin-care ranges these days: **Comfrey, Calendula (Marigold)** and **Chamomile**. This extraordinary trio, which can be grown with ease in any garden, have unique powers to soften, soothe, protect and heal the skin.

Comfrey promotes the growth or regeneration of skin tissue throughout the body, including that of the connective tissue vital to firm, youthful skin.

Marigold, or Calendula, will promptly clear up any infection of the skin; it is equally potent against fungal, viral or bacterial infection. Another great healer, it works by countering inflammation, and by its mild astringency. It is also useful for chapped skin, or thread veins.

Chamomile soothes, heals, combats inflammation and stimulates cell regeneration. German Chamomile – *Matricaria chamomilla* – is the variety most widely used in skin treatment; it is rich in a fatty substance called azulene, which has extraordinary healing, anti-bacterial and anti-inflammatory powers.

All three can be made up into a strong infusion, steeped covered, strained, cooled and used as a facial rinse morning and evening. Keep it in the fridge for no more than 24 hours, and use up the rest in a bath. Or use these herbs in a facial sauna (see p.78). Try using a handful of the fresh leaves or flowers to make your own oil; follow the directions for making an infused oil on p.144. (See also The Skin, p.73, for the uses of these herbs in soothing and healing skin disorders.)

TO MAKE OYLE OF CAMOMILE
Take oyle a pint and a halfe and 3oz
camomile flowers dryed one day after they
be gathered. Then put the oyle and flowers
in a glasse and stop the mouth close and set
it into the sun by the space of 40 days.
The Good Housewife's Handbook, *1588*
(cit. A Garden of Herbs,
Eleanor Sinclair Rohde)

Oranges are great for your skin. Take the pulp of a whole Orange and process or blend it to a smooth purée; apply it all over your face, neck, hands (newly washed). Leave on for about 20 minutes, then wash off with tepid water. Apart from the lovely fresh tingle, your skin will have absorbed some of the vitamin C *and* the beta-carotene, and the complex of bioflavonoids called vitamin P which strengthen the tiny capillaries, protecting you from unsightly broken veins.

To freshen a greasy skin, add 1 part of freshly squeezed Orange juice to 4 parts of **Rose Water** or distilled **Witch-Hazel**, both of which can be bought cheaply at your local chemist. Use it as a tonic.

Grated Orange rind and yoghurt is a good moisturizing and reviving mask that will put a glow back into your skin.

Orange flower water – available at chemists – has some of the rejuvenating properties of the Orange: it is a lovely freshener, good for young or problem skins.

Floral vinegars for skin care were particularly popular with Victorian women, who used them as a body-splash after the bath, or – well diluted – as a tonic for their complexions. You would not expect vinegar to leave your skin soft and smooth, but that is exactly what it does – used with care; it restores the natural acid balance of your skin, which can be stripped away by soap or alcohol-based lotions. Use red **Rose** petals for a beautifully-coloured Rose vinegar. Gather the petals early in the morning, clip off the white petal bases, and put a couple of handfuls of them in a wide-mouthed jar. Cover with a good white wine or cider vinegar, and macerate for 3 weeks; then strain out the vinegar and bottle. You can dilute it with the addition of an equal part of Rose water. Then use it diluted – like all toilet vinegars – 1 part to 4 parts of water.

Lavender vinegar was another great favourite, made by steeping the freshly gathered flowering tops in white wine vinegar for a week, shaking the bottle from time to time. Lavender is soothing and antiseptic for a troubled skin, helps balance over-active sebaceous glands, and stimulates the growth of healthy new skin cells.

AROMATIC TOILET VINEGAR
Dry a good quantity of rose leaves,
lavender flowers and jasmine flowers.
Weigh them, and to every 4 oz of rose
leaves (petals), allow 1 oz each of lavender
and jasmine. Mix them well together, pour
over them 2 pints of white vinegar, and
shake well, then add ½pint of rosewater
and shake again. Stand aside for ten days,
then strain and bottle.
A Modern Herbal
(Mrs M. Grieve, 1931)

Cider vinegar is one of the cheapest cosmetics there is. You can use it diluted 1 part to 6 of mineral or ordinary water.

Fizzing mineral water is a terrific reviver for the skin. On a long flight once I went for a wash and freshen-up – only to discover that there was no water coming out of the tap. I told a passing steward, who brought me a bottle of sparkling mineral water. I happily washed my hands in it and splashed it all over my face – a wonderful tonic for skin dehydrated by a long flight.

Spritzing your face is another lovely way to freshen up. Evian water comes packaged in aerosol (environmentally-friendly) spray cans. After spritzing, allow to dry for a couple of minutes, then blot off the excess and apply moisturizer; this will help hold the water in your skin, keeping it moist.

For a home-made spritzer, buy a small plant-mister and keep it for your personal use. You can spritz with any bottled spring water. Aromatherapist Julia Lawless suggests a fragrant alternative. Using spring or de-ionized water, add 30 drops of essential oil to every 100ml/3½floz of water. Leave closed for a few days in the dark, then filter through coffee paper. The oil will be blotted up by the paper; its therapeutic properties and aroma will be left in the water. Try **Lavender, Bergamot** or **Geranium** for an oily skin; **Rose, Neroli** or **Jasmine** for dry or normal skin; or **Grapefruit** for dull congested skin.

Benzoin is the resinous gum of the *Styrax benzoin* tree, growing in Java and Malaysia. The simple tincture is sold by chemists; add 6-8 drops to a cupful of the distilled water you use in your spritzer to help chapped or dry skin, and close pores. Or add a splash of cooling, astringent **Witch-Hazel** to your spritzing water, if your skin is inclined to be greasy.

Your morning cleansing milk could be just that – ordinary milk; it is fine for dry or normal skins. Use it as you would any ordinary cleansing lotion, on pads of cottonwool, using a tonic or freshener afterwards. Milk is a cleanser for oily skin, too, which will benefit from its tonic and nutritive properties. But 'cut' it first with a splash of *eau-de-cologne*, Witch-Hazel, or tincture of Benzoin.

Avoid soap for your face, unless it is a specially formulated complexion soap with the correct pH balance. Most soaps have a pH of at least 7, often as high as 10, which will strip away the acid mantle of your skin, leaving it feeling taut and dry.

Steer clear of alcohol-based lotions, too; they are very drying, which is not beneficial even to oily skins.

Generations of women have used **Sweet Almond** oil to soften dry skin and soothe away blemishes. Two or 3 times a week, film your face and neck with Almond oil; leave it on for 25 minutes before tissuing it off. Then give your face a refreshing splash with a toilet vinegar. This is also good for soothing skin that has been explosed to strong sun, wind, or freezing cold.

Add 2 or 3 drops of your favourite essential oil to the bottle, to enhance its effect and its fragrance. Try **Chamomile, Lavender** or

---

The oil of Almonds makes smooth the hands and face of delicate persons, and cleanseth the skin from all spots and pimples.

The Herball or Generall Histoire of Plantes
(John Gerard, 1633)

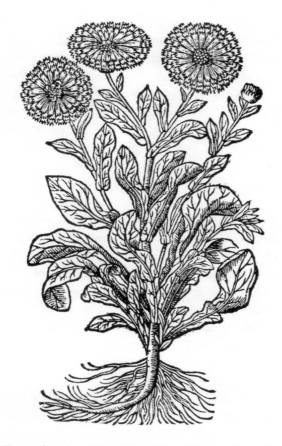

Rose for dry skin, **Neroli** or **Clary Sage** for older skin.

A facial sauna is a good start to a deep-cleansing treatment for your face. It opens up the pores, stimulates the circulation and helps the skin sweat out wastes. If your skin is dry to normal, give it an occasional steam, followed by a bracing and tonic facial (see p.79 for suggestions). Oily or blemished skins can take a weekly sauna. Do not steam your face, though, if your skin is highly sensitive, blotchy, easily irritated, or if you have little broken veins.

The benefits of this facial sauna can be boosted by adding a strong infusion of herbs. Depending on what you have to hand, try purifying and healing **Lavender**, antiseptic **Sage** or **Lemon** peel, healing **Rosemary** or Mari-

gold. **Yarrow** is tonic and astringent; **Rosemary** stimulates circulation; **Chamomile** and Lavender soothe and heal troubled skin. **Peppermint** or **Elderflower** have a stimulating, firming effect; **Fennel** is great for cleansing, **Mallow** for softening, **Cornflower** for refreshing. Mallow, Marigold and Sage are particularly good for problem skins, Comfrey and **Borage** flowers for dry skin.

To give yourself a facial sauna, put a generous handful of your chosen herb in a glass or enamel pan, off the heat. Pour in 500ml/¾ pint of boiling water, cover the pan, and let it infuse for 10 minutes. Then put the pan on the stove, and bring it gently back to near-boiling point. Take it off – have towels ready – and steam your face, not too close, in a tent of towel to keep the steam in, for 5–10 minutes.

Blot your face dry, splash it with **Rose** water, Orange-flower water, Elderflower water, or a diluted toilet vinegar, and stay indoors for an hour or so.

You can use essential oil instead of herbs by adding 3-4 drops to steaming-hot water. **Bergamot** or **Lavender** for oily skin; **Chamomile, Ylang-Ylang** or **Jasmine** for dry skin, **Lavender** or **Cedarwood** for blemished skin.

For oily skins, take a tablespoon each of **Chamomile** flowers and **Thyme**, add to a litre/1¾ pints of water and simmer covered for 10 minutes. Strain, cool, and use as a face wash. Swab it on liberally, and let it dry on your skin – perhaps while you have a bath, into which you tip the rest of the infusion; this will help counter fatigue.

Rub a freshly-cut **Potato** over your skin, leave to dry for 10 minutes, then rinse off. It helps slough off dead cells, heals and nourishes.

For oily skins, an **Oatmeal** scrub will leave

your skin clear, fresh and silky soft. Oatmeal supplies lots of nutrients to your skin, including B-complex vitamins and calcium. Buy the colloidal Oatmeal specially prepared for cosmetic use; use it daily mixed with water, to remove the last traces of grime or make-up from your skin. To enhance its effect, you can mix it with **Rose** water, or **Cider** vinegar, or **Lemon** juice added to the water. An Oatmeal scrub is good for blemished skins, too.

Or make up an Oatmeal mask with a tablespoonful of colloidal Oatmeal, 2-3 drops of Lemon juice and a spoonful of cream. Add ½ teaspoon of brewer's yeast for extra nourishment. This will feed and soften your skin, and stimulate cellular metabolism.

When you make a herbal tisane, use a couple of spoonfuls of it to give your skin a drink too. **Peppermint** is an excellent tonic for oily skin, pepping it up before you apply make-up for an evening out. **Chamomile** calms congested or reddened skin. **Limeflowers** revitalize your skin and calm sunburn.

A face-mask or facial can work wonders for your skin if you want to look good in the evening after a long, draining day. If you have time, steam your skin first with an infusion of **Rosemary** or **Thyme** to open your pores and stimulate the circulation. Otherwise, just clean your skin thoroughly. Then put on your favourite music, spread one of the following facial or masks over your face and neck, lie down and relax for 15 minutes. Rinse off with tepid water, then freshen with **Rose** water. Let your skin rest for at least an hour, if possible, before putting on make-up.

Maurice Messegue suggests crushing a handful of fresh herbs or flowers in a cupful of fresh cream, adding the yolk of an egg for dry skins, or the whipped white for greasy. Try **Borage** flowers, **Rose** petals, **Lavender** flowers, **Sage** and **Violets**. Or add **Carrot** juice, crushed **Cucumber** or **Pumpkin** flesh, **Watercress** or grated **Potato**.

Carrot finely grated into Olive oil for use as a face-mask is an Italian favourite for dry and delicate skins; it is particularly nourishing.

Pure **Grape** juice, or peeled and crushed fresh **Grapes**, will help give your skin a soft springy look.

Whipped egg-white combined with **Aloe Vera** gel makes a firming mask for sagging skin. Aloe Vera is astringent and soothing at the same time; it contains a polysaccharide that helps skin retain moisture; it also promotes the growth of healthy new skin cells.

If you make mayonnaise, do not throw away the whites of the egg. Whip them up and add a teaspoon of **Lemon** juice; this is good to brace and firm oily and greasy skin.

Honey softens rough skin, and helps it retain moisture. The bees have already added herbs for you; **Clover** honey is lovely for ageing, sallow skin; **Limeflower** honey is purifying and calming.

Almond meal – you can buy ground Almonds in any supermarket – heals and nourishes the skin; make up a mask with **Rose** or **Orange** flower water or milk.

Try blending a couple of slices of **Apple** with 2 teaspoonfuls of **Lemon** juice, to moisturize and stimulate your skin.

For tired and jaded skins, a lovely summertime tonic is the crushed flesh of ripe **Cherries**.

Peach flesh pressed over dry or ageing skin, left on for 20 minutes or so, will help regenerate tissues and restore the acid balance.

History comes full circle; we still laugh about the paranoia of Victorian and Edwardian women, who never stirred into the sunshine without a parasol to protect their faces. Today, we are being strongly warned against the ageing and wrinkling effect of too much sunshine (not to mention the risk of skin cancer). Few women, on the other hand, worry about a freckle or two. If you do, however, there are a number of classic remedies for gently bleaching them out of your skin. Soothe **Almond** oil into your skin afterwards to counteract their drying effect:

Try grated **Horseradish** mixed with yogurt, or steeped in milk, or **Cider** vinegar.

Pure **Lemon** juice, painted on neat, or mixed with ⅓ of rum, may help.

Elderflower water was popular with seventeenth-century beauties.

For skins which have had an overdose of sunshine, add 2-3 drops of **Chamomile** to a small bottle of **Avocado** or **Almond** oil; use every day for a week or so. Or try **Marigold** oil: leave for 20 minutes, blot off and freshen with

To help a face that is red or pimpled. Dissolve common Salt in the iuyce of Lemmons, and with a linnen cloth pat the patient's face that is full of heat or pimples. It cureth in a few dressings.

Delights for Ladies
(Sir Hugh Plat)

diluted **Cider** vinegar.

Another useful remedy for sunburn is this Victorian **Cucumber** lotion. Chop up a Cucumber and squeeze out the juice with a Lemon-squeezer. Mix this with a quantity of glycerine and Rose water mixed together in equal parts. Add 8-10 drops of simple tincture of Benzoin, to promote the healing effect of this lotion, and to act as an antioxidant. Keep this lotion in your fridge, for up to a week.

HANDS AND FEET

Our hands are almost always on show, our feet almost never; but both hands and feet are particularly hard-working parts of us, in their different ways, and need all the care and attention we can spare time to give them.

When my mother was a young girl, she and her sisters were taught to come down to the drawing-room to meet visitors with their hands held high above their heads. Lowering them as they opened the door and walked in, they were able to offer a beautifully pale and bloodless hand in greeting.

To keep their hands soft and pale, women invariably wore gloves out of doors; in my first job – working for *Vogue* – I spent fortunes on kid gloves, *de rigueur* for the staff of a glossy

magazine at the time. Most of us go gloveless today, however, except in the depths of winter. So our hands are exposed to all weathers – plus dust and grime.

A huge range of chemicals in household cleaners are another hazard. Hands that wash dishes without rubber gloves on will not be soft and smooth (whatever the advertisements say). Some of the substances used in detergents, washing-powders, washing-up liquids, polishes, and cleaners generally can be very irritant to the skin. Housewives' Dermatitis is familiar to skin specialists. Simply pulling the washing out of the machine and hanging it out to dry – a chore for which who would think of pulling on rubber gloves? – can be enough to irritate the skin, if you are sensitive to a particular ingredient in the washing-powder. Wearing rubber gloves for long spells may not do your hands much good either, since sweat will be trapped inside them.

Excessive heat can produce dry chapped hands, too. And constant washing of your hands certainly will – it dries out the skin.

Much of this wear and tear is unavoidable. Fortunately, there is a wealth of simple plant-derived ingredients – many of them on sale cheaply from your local chemist, others usually to hand in your kitchen – which will help you keep your hands soft and smooth, in spite of everything.

Almonds or Almond oil turn up in all the best recipes, ancient and modern, for hand-care. You can make a soft paste of ground Almonds and a little Rose water; spread it on your hands when you have a little leisure, and leave it on for as long as possible. When you rinse it off, smooth in a little hand-cream at once. In her book *Feed your Face*, Dian Dincin Buchman gives a recipe she adapted from a more complicated one used by her grandmother: moisten Almond meal with a little milk or Almond oil, and make a paste with the yolk of an egg, a few drops of Cider vinegar and a large spoonful of pure honey. 'I apply this to my hands and cover them with cotton gloves.' (If you want to keep this on all night, incidentally, buy a large size of those thin plastic gloves sold for hospital use, and wear them *over* the cotton gloves, or your sheets will be a mess.)

Rosewater used by itself can be drying; added to other creams or liquids, though, it helps keep in moisture. Mix equal parts of Rosewater and **Glycerin**, both of which you can buy from a chemist; Glycerin is a humectant, and together they will stop moisture evaporating from your skin.

Dry, cracked and sore hands may be a case of eczema or dermatitis, or a local allergic reaction, or even – as once in my own case, shrewdly diagnosed by my herbalist – a flare-up of *herpes*. If the condition persists despite endless creams, lotions and oils, you will need expert advice from a dermatologist, or a qualified herbal practitioner or aromatherapist, but try any of the following first.

A 500-year-old recipe 'To Whiten and Smooth the Hands' was quoted in the US bestseller, *The Natural Formula Book for Home and Yard*. Use of it, say the authors, cured and healed within days the painfully cracked hands of a woman who had suffered agonies from them for 3 years. Here is the recipe:

25g/1oz ground Almonds; 1 egg, beaten; ¼oz ground Comfrey root; a tablespoon Honey. Combine the Almonds, egg, Comfrey root and Honey, and mix them with your hands. (Keep this mixture in the fridge.) At night, coat your hands with it, and pull on an old pair of kid gloves, if you have them – they will not leak – or a pair of cotton gloves. Repeat nightly for a week, rinse your hands (and the gloves) in the morning and apply a cream or lotion. After a week, repeat once a week, for a month, and then monthly.

A number of essential oils are healing and soothing: **Benzoin, Chamomile** and **Lavender** among them. Decant 50 ml/1½floz of **Almond** or **Olive** oil into a little bottle; add 25-30 drops of one of these, pierce and squeeze in a vitamin E capsule (200 or 400 international units strength) and shake thoroughly. Warm the bottle under a running hot tap before use, so that the oil is nice and warm. Give your hands a gentle bedtime massage, soothing and rubbing the oil well into the skin and around the nails. Then towel off the surplus, and do not wash your hands again till morning. Some people even wear cotton gloves to keep the skin supple!

If the oil treatment does not work, buy a simple, unperfumed cream, or a plain hand-cream, and add the essential oils to it: 25-30 drops to 125g/5oz of cream, plus the contents of a vitamin E capsule.

Fungal infections around the nails can be both persistent and painful, with reddened sore cuticles, and a slight discharge. If unchecked, the nail will eventually become ridged and deformed and may have to be removed. French doctors have had great success using twice-daily applications of pure **Tea Tree** oil. The treatment may have to be persevered with for several weeks.
N.B. Some people find Tea Tree oil irritant to their skin. Try it in a patch test first, and use it diluted 1-3 in a bland oil for the first few treatments, until you are sure you are not reacting to it.

To strengthen nails, soak them in a strong infusion of dried **Horsetail**. 1 tbsp to 500ml/¾ pint of water, infused for 30 minutes. Horsetail is rich in silicon, a natural constituent of nails, hair and collagen.

Pure **Lemon** juice is softening and whitening too. Keep halves of Lemon after you have squeezed the juice from them; scrabble your fingers in them. Do not throw away the skins of **Avocados** either, until you have sleeked the insides over your hands – a wonderfully rich, creamy treatment.

We give our feet a hard time. We squash them into tight-fitting shoes, encase them day-long in synthetic fabrics through which they cannot breathe properly, compel them to support us for hours on end, and pound hard city pavements with them.

Corns, callouses, bunions, blisters, verrucas, burning feet, smelly feet, athlete's foot: these are among the consequences of the cavalier way we treat our feet. Then we complain about them, 'My feet are killing me,' we say.

Unfortunately, it is hard to take feet problems seriously. Corns and bunions can be a bit of a joke, until you suffer from them.

Pampering your feet is an enlightened form of self-interest; so start pampering now – they will repay you in aces.

Wear comfortable shoes, leather if possible, on all but the rarest of special occasions. If you always wear skirts and synthetic tights, get into the trouser habit and give your feet a break in pure cotton socks at least some of the time. Pamper them when you have time with alternating hot, cold and scented footbaths, to get the circulation moving in cramped toes. Putting your feet up rests you as much as them.

Corns are a defence mechanism your feet resort to when life gets tough for them in ill-fitting shoes; the skin hardens, and gradually the patch of callous becomes a little plug of extra-hard skin burrowing down into your toe. There are plenty of country remedies for corns that are well worth trying, if only to avoid a visit to the chiropodist.

Before you go to bed, soak your feet in warm water to which you have added a handful of Epsom salts. Afterwards, massage your feet, especially the corns, with a little **Castor** oil. Sleep in cotton socks to spare your sheets.

Here is a poet's remedy: the petals of the white **Lily** macerated in a good white wine vinegar for a week. Strain and swab the corns night and morning with this.

Common **Ivy** is a favourite country remedy, soothing and comforting; soak some of the leaves for a day or two in **Cider** vinegar, or for 2-3 hours in pure **Lemon** juice. Then give your feet a good long soak in very hot water. Apply 2-3 leaves to the corn, and tape securely into place. Repeat this until the corns are soft enough to lift out.

Garlic is another tried and tested remedy. At night-time, circle the corn with a corn plaster, then fill the hole above the corn with crushed Garlic. Tape over and round it. Repeat until the corn softens and comes out.

Using the same corn-plaster technique, fill the hole with crushed fresh **Radish** or Radish juice, or with freshly-pressed Lemon juice.

Like Aloe Vera, the plump leaves of the **Houseleek** are filled with a thick juice under the thin skin; it has been used by country people in some of the same ways, for similar problems. For corns, pick a strong young leaf from a young rosette and wash it carefully. Peel one side and apply it to the corn, taping it into place. Repeat night and morning till the corn is soft enough to remove.

Fungal infections of the feet and toenails respond to **Tea Tree** oil (see above, Hands, p.82). Add 10 drops of Tea Tree oil to a hot salted footbath and soak for at least 10 minutes. The fungus responsible for these infections thrive in the warm moist skin between toes, so it is vital to keep feet clean and dry, and to make sure they get as much air as possible.

Try a strong decoction of antiseptic **Thyme** or **Sage**. Repeat regularly till the infection clears.

To keep your feet soft, supple and free of infection, take a footbath 2-3 times a week in warm water to which you have added a tablespoonful of **Lemon** juice or a couple of table-

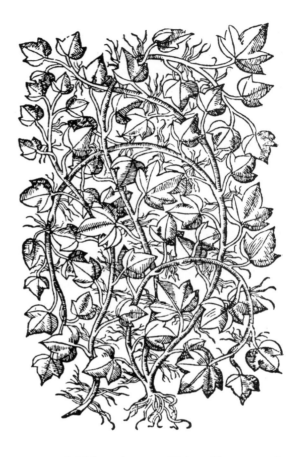

spoons of **Cider** vinegar. This will restore the acid mantle of the skin.

Verrucas and warts – the result of viral activity – can also be treated with Tea Tree oil; put a single drop on the centre, and cover with a plaster. Renew regularly. If this does not work within a week, crush a clove of **Garlic** and apply in a corn plaster, as above. The milky juice squeezed out from the stem of the **Celandine** or the **Dandelion** is another country cure.

All the **Mints** are a cooling, refreshing treat for tired feet. 4-5 drops of **Peppermint** oil in a tepid footbath is one way to enjoy the Mint treatment. Or you can infuse a couple of Peppermint teabags for at least 10 minutes, then add the tea to your footbath. If your feet become swollen easily, and you have a long evening in party shoes ahead of you, Danièle Ryman suggests massaging the soles of your feet first with a little oil-mixture – 10 drops of Peppermint oil added to a couple of teaspoons of **Grapeseed** oil (a particularly bland, fast-penetrating oil).

Young ballet students, who are apt to have little spare cash, use ordinary cold Tea, which is cooling and astringent.

All ballet dancers, points out Patricia Davis, tend to suffer from cracked skin on their poor overworked feet: they use Friar's Balsam from a chemist – compound tincture of **Benzoin** – to paint on to the painful sores, preventing further damage.

One of the most embarrassing complaints is feet that sweat a lot, and inevitably become smelly. This is because your skin – nicknamed 'the third kidney' since it is also a major organ of elimination – is getting an overload (see Cleansing, p.89).

Make sure that your feet are kept as dry, as cool and as fresh as possible. Wear *only* cotton socks. If possible, avoid wearing shoes for two days in a row. Walk around barefoot or in sandals at home whenever possible. At bedtime, give your feet a footbath to which you add 8-10 drops of **Tea Tree** oil. Dry thoroughly, particularly between the toes. Footbaths with a good splash of **Cider** vinegar are helpful, too. Sweaty feet have often lost their healthy acid count, and need to be switched back into it using these methods.

REMEDIES

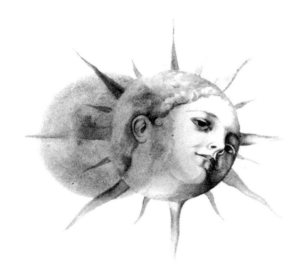

INTRODUCTION

Most of the herbalists whose work has inspired and delighted me grew up with a mother or grandmother who was herself an enthusiastic amateur herbalist. They recall being dosed with herbs as children, seeing the bundles of useful herbs drying in the kitchen, watching remedies being concocted, being shown the growing plants so that they themselves could learn to identify them.

In the small Cotswold village where I was born and grew up, there may have been such experts around, but there were none in my family. The only herbal remedy I remember using was the classic Dock leaf for a Nettle sting. Otherwise we used patent medicines or sent for the doctor like everyone else.

As I mentioned in the Foreword, it was only many years later that I first began to discover for myself how effective herbs could be in treating the minor medical problems of a young family.

I am not a trained practitioner, and do not presume to offer advice for serious disorders. But as every wife and mother learns over the years, there are numerous minor health problems which she may be called on to deal with and if possible relieve: hangovers; bouts of 'flu; childhood fevers; sore throats; coughs, earaches; burns; sunburn; sleeplessness; indigestion and diarrhoea among them.

Most of them are what doctors call 'self-limiting'; in other words they usually clear up of their own accord within 3 or 4 days. Meanwhile, loved ones are restless, uncomfortable or in pain; it is the most natural of instincts to want to make them better, sooner.

Some of these problems, even the minor ones, may not go away, however; untreated, they may worsen and become serious. The cough not dealt with may develop into bronchitis; the diarrhoea become chronic, or more severe; the sleeplessness habitual; the earache a massive infection. The doctor will then need to be called, and powerful drugs prescribed. In the end, it may be weeks before normal buoyant health is restored, when a simple, harmless herbal remedy and a little common sense might have sorted out the problem in its early stages.

There is no Herbe, nor weede, but God hath gyven vertue to them, to help man.
The Fyrste Boke of the Introduction of Knowledge
(Andrew Boorde, 1490-1549)

Professional herbalists are often critical of amateurs such as myself, denouncing what they call 'the symptomatic approach'. Herbs are *not* just gentle drugs to deal with a symptom and make it go away, they maintain. They are quite right, when talking about serious health problems, or chronic illness. There is very little point in spending time and money concocting herbal remedies for health problems which result from the way we live, eat, work and relax. If our lifestyle is making us ill, all the herbs in the world will not make us better without some other effort on our part.

If you give someone with a stomach ulcer something to make the pain go away temporarily, without treating the causes, or if you give a soothing digestive remedy to someone who gobbles lunch at their desk and has three strong Scotches before dinner, or if you take Ginger tea to relieve the nausea of pregnancy without stopping to ask why you keep getting nauseated – you are indeed guilty of the symptomatic approach. In the long run you will not help the problem.

The professional herbalist, by contrast, would want to know *why* the ulcer, the indigestion, or the nausea is happening in the first place, correct the lifestyle mistakes which gave rise to them, and treat the systemic weakness and damage which has resulted. He or she may seem strangely unconcerned about the particular aches or pains which brought about the visit. This holistic approach is undoubtedly the best and most effective way to approach our health problems.

We must be realistic, however. Only a small minority of people will consult their local herbalist; and most people are not in the least interested to know why they have an ulcer, or arthritis, or recurrent headaches. If you cannot give them something to ease the pain or relieve the symptoms, they will go to the chemist or their sympathetic GP for drug treatment which does.

In my view, even the 'symptomatic' herbal remedy is preferable to the drug in these cases, and it will probably be just as effective at giving temporary relief for pain and discomfort. Unlike many prescription drugs, it will be mild enough to have no damaging side-effects. It is also likely to act as a tonic to the affected system, since almost every herb in common domestic use has a number of beneficial 'side-effects'. This is exactly how so many women have used herbal remedies through the centuries.

Herbs can do a great deal more for us, however, whether in the form of marvellous medicinal plants, or as what we normally consider only as foodstuffs which we eat every day. We can learn to use them not just as curative, but as preventive medicine.

Leon Binet, the great French authority on plant medicine, described herbal *tisanes* as, 'real elements of health'. The following three were his favourites: an infusion of Blackcurrant leaves in the morning; an infusion of Peppermint at noon; an infusion of Limeflowers at night. A diuretic regime, it might be objected? 'Perhaps,' he would reply. 'But also a detoxifying regime, a tonic regime, a calming regime.'

'Herbs can be used freely and safely as part of one's lifestyle without thinking of them as "medicines",' says David Hoffman, in the introduction to his book *The New Holistic Herbal*.

For specific health needs, their best use would be preventative – to prevent specific problems appearing. There are specific herbs which strengthen and tone specific organs and systems. These may be used where a tendency towards illness is recognized but no overt disease is present. By using herbs it may well be possible to overcome any weakness.

If your lungs are your weakness, for example, you might substitute for tea or coffee a herbal infusion of Mullein or White Horehound, Sage or Rosemary. It would also make sense to include plenty of the cleansing vegetables of the Crucifer family in your diet – Watercress, Cabbage, Horseradish, Radishes, Turnips, Broccoli as well as Garlic, Onions and Leeks.

If your circulation is poor, and you have a tendency to varicose veins, piles, chilblains or little broken capillaries in your skin, choose tisanes of Angelica root, Hawthorn flowers or Yarrow; use Cayenne pepper or Ginger in your seasoning, and eat Buckwheat, Garlic and Seaweed.

Even if you develop a specific health prob-

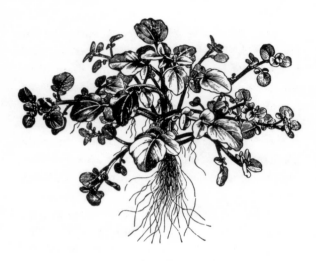

lem for which you have consulted a doctor and are following a course of drugs – bronchitis, a stomach ulcer, or high blood pressure – there are mild herbal teas you can safely take at the same time; these will act to improve your general resistance during the course of treatment.
N.B. Herbs can be powerful medicine, however, and amateurs should not attempt to treat serious health problems themselves. If you had a severe heart condition, for instance, it would not occur to you to hunt through the pharmacist's shelves and pick out a drug you felt might be appropriate, even if this were possible. Neither should you attempt to select the herbs to treat that condition, which is a matter for an experienced herbalist.

This is especially true if you are already taking prescribed drugs, when a medicinal herb taken at the same time might interfere with their activity. Let your doctor know of any herbal remedy you propose to take at the same time as any drugs he has prescribed.

How do you know when your health problem is too serious for amateur herbal prescribing? In a thoughtful article for *The Herbalist*, Simon Mills lays down a good general rule,

'. . . never treat an *extreme* symptom of any sort, or one that *perseveres* unduly: anything that fails to respond to treatment must similarly be referred to a professional.' (There are many trained herbal practitioners in Britain – see Useful Addresses, p.158.)

In such circumstances your choice of herb might actually worsen rather than improve your condition. For instance, chronic constipation can be the result either of lack of tone in the gut walls, or the exact opposite – too much tension in the muscles that should keep things moving. Each condition needs a completely different herbal approach, and the wrong one would aggravate matters instead of improving them.

Within these limits, the regular use of mild safe herbs can only be of benefit. Most of the herbs recommended in this book are mild and safe, and can be taken regularly for weeks, months, or even a lifetime. In cases where this is not so, I have noted the fact.

There is one outstanding way in which herbs can help to improve your general health. Use them as wonderful, systemic cleansers and detoxifiers, at the end of winter perhaps; after the over-indulgence of a holiday period; or at times when you feel run-down or off-colour.

The next section is devoted to this cleanisng process.
N.B. As in Part 2, the first time a herb is mentioned as a remedy it is written in bold type.

The country people in this our Island do make use of Kitchen Physic; and common experience tells that they who least employ apothercaries' physick do live freest from all manner of infirmities.
Secret Miracles of Nature, *1658*
(cit. Fernie, Kitchen Physic*)*

CLEANSING/*LE DRAINAGE*

The French have a word for it: *Le Drainage* – the thorough and efficient elimination of the body's wastes.

Our bodies offload an amazing amount of rubbish every day: about 1500ml of urine, about 800ml of sweat, solid rubbish in the form of stools, and gaseous junk breathed out through our lungs. Some of it is metabolic waste produced by our bodies in the course of normal existence – dead cells and other debris. Some is what is left of the food we eat after digestion. Increasingly we have to deal with toxic wastes – food additives, pesticides, drugs, inhaled chemicals from car exhausts and other pollutants.

Much of the processing happens in our digestive tracts. Everything we eat or drink is broken down and sorted out somewhere along the length of this vital piece of tubing with the help of the liver and kidneys. Nutrients – and many toxins too, unfortunately – are absorbed through the intestinal walls into the bloodstream, for circulation via the liver to wherever they are needed. The rest is for junking – most solids through the bowels, most liquids – filtered by the kidneys – through the bladder.

The body has two more regular channels of elimination, of which we are much less aware: the skin and the lungs. In 24 hours, we sweat through our skins about 800ml of liquid, just over a pint. Sweat has been compared to diluted urine, and it has much the same composition: urea and uric acid, the metabolic by-products of protein digestion, water and other debris. In a fever, our 24-hourly output can rise to as much as 3 litres.

The lungs turn their wastes into gases, which are then breathed out.

In normal health, our organs of detoxification and elimination – liver, kidneys, bowels, lungs, skin – carry out their task unaided by us. When the rubbish starts to pile up, however, and things get out of hand, the practised French *phytotherapeute* knows that it is time for a spot of *drainage*, a skilled and precise procedure. He will select a number of herbs – *les draineurs* – calculated to strengthen, tone and stimulate specific eliminative systems.

Naturopath Christopher Vasey, who practises at Montreux in Switzerland, has devoted an authoritative book to the subject, the *Manuel de Detoxication*. 'Le Drainage' he says, 'is not just excellent preventive medicine: it is a most effective treatment for illness in its own right.'

The fundamental assumption in Natural Medicine is that disease results when our body's wastes are not efficiently cleared. The first signs of trouble are fatigue, lethargy, depression, and a general lack of vitality. More problems arise when the body starts resorting to secondary, emergency elimination channels. Extra wastes are eliminated through the lungs in the form of mucus (a cold); or excess wax in the ear (and your child gets Glue Ear); or an unusually heavy monthly discharge.

Things are more serious when the body is forced to start stockpiling the waste it can no longer get rid of: bronchitis, gout or arthritis could be the result. Finally, the organs of elimination themselves reach crisis point, and jaundice or nephritis might be the consequence.

The common cold furnishes us with a good example of how the system works. Orthodox medicine insists that a cold is 'caught', the work of an unfriendly virus: Natural Medicine knows better.

Typically, a cold develops in winter, after you go out and get thoroughly chilled. What actually happens, though, is that in winter we take much less exercise, and eat heavier, richer food. As a result, our eliminative systems are already working overtime, without much help from us. That chilled-to-the-bone feeling is the last straw: the skin surface closes down and we sweat less so that the body can conserve heat; so one of our four eliminative channels is out of action. Where does all that waste go now? Out through the respiratory system, of course, in the form of mucus. As this piles up in our mucous membranes, it offers an excellent breeding ground for viruses, bacteria or fungi. Now we really have 'caught a cold'. Equally, a cold can be caught in summer, if your resistance is low.

The successful herbal way to stop the cold gettting into its stride is to go to bed with a hot drink, preferably plenty of Elderflower tea. *Any* hot drink will make you sweat a bit, and so get your skin functioning as an eliminative channel again. But Elderflower does more: not only diaphoretic – encouraging perspiration – it also acts on the kidneys to boost their eliminative action.

Treatment for toxic overload falls into two parts: elimination of the excess wastes and the strengthening of the weakened organs.

French phytotherapists select herbs especially tailored to each eliminative system – diuretics, laxatives, sudorifics, diaphoretics, cholagogues and others. Some of these herbs are powerful tonics or stimulants, with highly specific actions. *Le Drainage* calls for expert diagnosis and prescription. It is possible to overstimulate organs so that you weaken them instead of strengthening, and it takes experience to avoid mistakes of this kind.

There are a number of common foods and herbs, however, which will not only encourage the elimination of wastes, but will also gently tone and nourish specific organs; they may strengthen and cleanse your whole system at the same time.

Most of them are herbs that have featured in the spring cures of country medicine down the centuries, as Green drinks taken to give the system a spring-clean, and get you off to a new start after the heavy, over-eating, months of winter. Others are Wild Foods such as Nettles and Dandelions, that country people regularly added to their diet, brewed up into teas or turned into homebrewed wines and beers.

If you have skin or digestive problems, recurrent bronchitis, arthritis or rheumatism, or even just a general sense of congestion, low energy and poor vitality, try the Cleansing Cure.

Essential to any *Drainage* programme is a diet trimmed of the major waste-producers: milk products; sugar; excess protein or fat; and additive-laden processed foods, biscuits, cakes, sweets and chocolate. Take plenty of exercise, and get lots of fresh air.

Study the indications below for each of your main eliminative systems; work out which may be giving you problems, and start adding the suggested foods to your diet. Many of the herbs suggested are foodstuffs as much as medicine. (See the end of this section for information on individual herbs useful to the eliminative systems.) Most of them, too, have a broad-spectrum action, cleansing and rejuvenating throughout the body. They are all mild herbs which can be taken over days without risk. Which eliminative system needs particular support? Here are some clues.

Intestines Signs of trouble: Constipation, 'Gas' and 'wind' produced by half-digested food fermenting or putrefying in the intestinal tract.

Constipation has many causes, but overload can be one of them.

Remedy Eat plenty of wholegrains, fruit and vegetables for fibre. Every evening, put 3-4 carefully-washed Figs or Prunes to soak in a bowl of water overnight. Eat them slowly, fasting, in the morning, and drink the water. Or drink Lettuce tea – 75g/3oz of Lettuce simmered for 30 minutes in a litre of water; take 3 cupfuls a day.

Liver Signs of trouble: Indigestion, nausea, a furred tongue, a bloated stomach.

Remedy Include Blackcurrants, Apples, Grapes, Celery, Artichokes, Chicory, Carrots, Olives, Olive oil, Parsley, Dandelions in your diet. Drink Rosemary tea or a decoction of Burdock.

Kidneys Signs of trouble: scanty, or dark-coloured, or cloudy or strong-smelling urine.

Remedy Fennel. Leeks. Onions. Cabbage – raw. Nettles. Take Plantain.

Skin Signs of trouble: Congested, blotchy, muddy skin, with black- or white-heads; pimples; boils – a sign of overworked or even blocked sebaceous glands – which can result from overload, as well as an unbalanced diet. Boils and abscesses are ways in which the body makes an extra outlet for rubbish, signs of serious overload.

Remedy Stimulate elimination through your skin by skin-brushing; brush yourself from toes to neck with long sweeping, upward strokes, using a natural bristle brush. Do it first thing in the morning, then have a quick cold sponge-down followed by a tepid wash. Take lots of exercise. Drink Elderflower tea, and take the following herbs: Burdock, Heart's ease (see Skin, p.120), and Blackcurrant leaves (see Tea-Time, p.50).

Lungs Signs of trouble: Stuffed-up or runny nose, clogged and painful sinuses, catarrh.

Remedy Eat plenty of Onions. Garlic. Watercress. Turnips. Horseradish. And take the following herbs: Plantain, Sage (note that Sage is best avoided in early pregnancy, or when breast-feeding).

Many of the herbs and foods are for more than one eliminative system.

THE HERBS

Burdock This is one of the great depurative herbs, assisting liver and kidneys, and helping clear dry scaly skin where dead cells have accumulated on the surface. Add 1 teaspoon of the chopped root to a cupful of water; bring to the boil and simmer 10-15 minutes. Take 3 times daily.

Dandelion Unless you are city-bound, a stroll through the countryside should supply all the Dandelion you can carry. Avoid plants that could have been contaminated by pesticide spraying or exhausts from passing cars. Pick out the young fresh leaves. Eat them in salads (see Wild Food p.00, for recipe); add to soups. Old-fashioned herbalists used to say that any herb which is particularly plentiful is sure to be especially valuable. Dandelions are a case in point, one of the greatest cleansers, detoxifiers and tonics in the plant kingdom.

Nettles These come to the rescue for both liver and kidneys, and are one of the great all-round spring-time cleansers. Add them to soups, stew them with Spinach or other greens (see Wild Food, p.00 for Nettle Pudding recipe). Only the young leaves are edible, in spring.

Plantain On a country walk, you can hardly help falling over this humble herb, which is a marvellous cleanser and purifier for the lungs, stomach and blood. Eat the young leaves chopped up in a salad: add them to soups, or blend them to green juices with Spinach, Watercress, Dandelion and other cleansing herbs. Add 25g/1oz of the herb to 600ml/1 pint of boiling water. Infuse for 20 minutes; take 3 cupfuls a day.

THE CIRCULATORY SYSTEM

Stout hearts are what we would all like to have. With a strong heart and good circulation, the whole body works better. Nutrients are delivered efficiently to first base; wastes regularly removed; many of the dismal afflictions of old age – poor digestion, varicose veins, failing sight, crepey skin, thinning hair – can be delayed for decades. If you are young in heart, you are young in body too.

What keeps the heart young and strong? Plenty of exercise. Good food. A relaxed attitude to life – however hard you work. Tranquillity. Fun. None of these is really beyond our reach, though some may be harder to achieve than others.

Eat and drink your way to a healthy heart (see What is Healthy Eating, p.22). A glass or two of good wine a day – but not more; not too much tea or coffee. Wholegrains are especially important: a nationwide switch from white bread to wholewheat could prevent enormous heart havoc. The bran and germs of grains like **Wheat, Rice** and **Oats** are rich in nutrients that our blood and arteries need, including fibre. A few of these nutrients are 're-placed' in refined flour but others are not; one of them is silicon.

Silicon is the second most common element on the planet, after oxygen; the human body contains around 1.4g – only slightly less than our supplies of vital zinc. Some is found in our blood, more in collagen throughout the body, and in hair, teeth and nails. Silicon keeps collagen young and healthy, which in turn maintains the suppleness and elasticity of your arteries. Researchers found that arteries thickened and hardened by arteriosclerosis had much lower amounts of silicon in them.

Rich sources of silicon are the skins of organically-grown fruits and vegetables, especially **Jerusalem Artichokes** and **Radishes**, and – particularly Oats. Other good sources are **Garlic, Pollen, Seaweeds** and sprouted seeds and grains, especially **Alfalfa**.

You read a lot about 'free radicals' in cosmetic advertisements these days; they damage and age the skin. Increasingly the whole ageing process, and much degenerative disease – including heart disease – is now seen as the result of free radical activity.

What are these alarming molecules? They are generated by metabolic activity in our bodies, formed naturally in the course of a wide range of metabolic processes essential to life. But things can get out of hand; free radicals are highly reactive, and in excess can combine with other molecules throughout the body to damage cell walls and membranes. The number of free radicals being generated in our bodies rises dramatically when we are exposed to pollution, radiation and strong sunshine; or when we absorb toxic substances such as tobacco smoke, alcohol, drugs, pesticide traces, synthetic additives, or food which has lost its freshness.

Fats, or lipids, are particularly attractive to free radicals; when they turn rancid after being exposed to oxygen, that is peroxidation at work. Thus the lipids, of which our cell membranes are largely formed, are ready victims to free radicals. Damage to the walls of capillaries, veins and arteries that can result in heart disease is one result.

Nature, as usual, has provided the answer. Excess free radicals are scavenged by substances called antioxidants, which are lavishly supplied in a healthy diet by fresh fruit and vegetables, in the form of vitamins A, C and E, and vitamin B2, some amino acids and many substances as yet unidentified. Recent research has revealed strong antioxidant activity in the essential oils of aromatic plants such as **Thyme, Sage** and **Oregano**. Enzymes such as superoxide dismutase in our bodies also act as antioxidants.

If our diets do not supply enough antioxidants, we are at risk. To make sure your diet does supply adequate quantities of them, turn to What is Healthy Eating, p.22.

Garlic is the King of Hearts. No man-made drug for heart problems can come anywhere near its efficacy or its versatility. Happily, many heart specialists are beginning to agree, so impressive is the evidence accumulating from many clinical trials. In an article in the *British Medical Journal* Michael Turner concluded that Garlic had demonstrated its worth in patients suffering from high blood pressure, high cholesterol, or a tendency to blood clotting, which can lead to thrombosis. Garlic lowered levels of low-density lipo-proteins (the kind associated with fatty deposits on arterial walls) and raised levels of high-density lipo-proteins (those which help keep our blood clear).

Drugs to control excess cholesterol or high blood pressure have to be taken year in, year out, and many doctors are uneasy about the potential side-effects. Garlic, however, can safely be consumed every day for a lifetime by almost anyone, preferably in its original raw form, rather than in the deodorized dried tablets that many people take. 'Much of the pharmacological activity of garlic is associated with the odorous compound allicin and its derivatives,' points out Michael Turner. 'Destroy the odour and effectiveness is reduced. . . . Let us not tamper unnecessarily with what nature provides.'

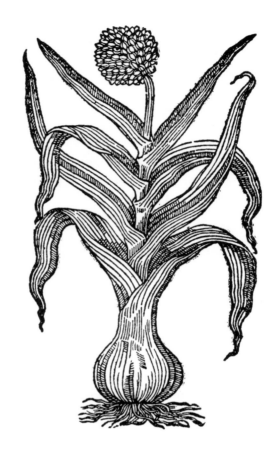

If you do worry about reeking of raw Garlic after adding a smear of it to your salad, you can always chew fresh Parsley, or Coffee beans.

There are many other food-medicines for the heart and circulatory system; among them **Leeks, Onions, Carrots, Oats, Barley**, and extra-virgin **Olive** oil.

N.B. Any of the herbs or food-medicines mentioned below can be used as suggested to keep your heart and arteries healthy. However, if you are aware of problems developing, you should consult your GP or a qualified herbalist straightaway: do not diagnose and prescribe for yourself. A herbalist will write a prescription personal to you, using as many as a dozen different herbs to help with different aspects of your problem. If you are under medical supervision, ask your doctor before adding a herbal drug to those he may have prescribed for you.

Herbalists use a number of herbs to deal with circulatory problems. High on their list is the **Hawthorn** berry. Sprigs of this plant used to be given to bridal couples in Ancient Greece, appropriately for this great friend of the heart. It has always been a highly-regarded herb, but it was not until the late nineteenth century that its extraordinary efficacy for heart problems began to be studied. The Hawthorn berry is a strong but gentle cardiac tonic; it will also lower high blood pressure, counter palpitations and arhythmias, and calm the agonies of *angina pectoris*, that sharp pain that signals heart disease. Its lack of toxicity makes it safe to take continuously over many years.

If I had a garden, I would plant a Hawthorn bush in it. But this is not an endangered plant, however, and you can probably find a bush safe from agricultural or Council spraying in your own neighbourhood. The bright red berries can be harvested in the autumn, and dried in the sun or in a very low oven. Crush them before making an infusion: 2 tsp of the berries to a cupful of water, infused for 20 minutes. Or you could try this Ayurvedic heart tonic. Simmer 12g/½oz of Hawthorn berries in 600ml/1 pint of water, together with a little powdered **Cinnamon** for 20 minutes. Take after meals, in wineglassful doses.

Just as common as Hawthorn, and almost as wide-ranging in its action, is the stinging **Nettle**. Nettles should feature regularly in the diet of those with heart problems, either eaten as a vegetable (see p.44) or drunk as a tea. Russian research has shown that a decoction of Nettles can improve heart function, while its rich iron content is a good tonic to help build blood.

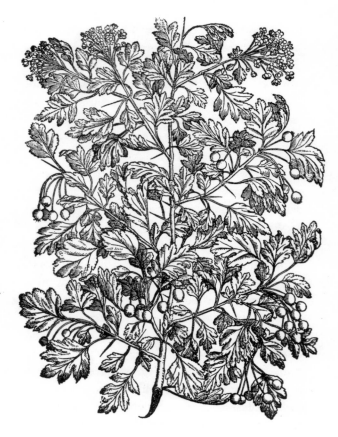

'Taken in conjunction with a good diet,' says herbalist Nalda Gosling, 'it will reduce the deposits in arteries and restore the elasticity of arterial walls. It has been found effective in thrombotic conditions'.

In Ayurvedic medicine, the warm spices have always been considered powerful and effective medicines. **Cinnamon** is believed to strengthen and harmonize blood flow; **Cardamom** stimulates the heart. **Cayenne** is another powerful heart stimulant; and **Ginger** is a general tonic for the heart and circulatory system.

Cayenne is widely – though not lavishly – used in the cookery of Italy, where the incidence of coronary disease is low. This is not surprising; Cayenne is recognized by herbalists as a tonic for the heart and the whole circulatory system, equally good for high or low blood pressure. But recent research has pinpointed a more specific protective action: Cayenne helps dissolve blood clots. In Thailand, where Cayenne features on almost every menu, cases of thrombosis are rare. They now know why. A Thai doctor conducted a study in a Bangkok hospital in which volunteers devoured noodles liberally spiced with Cayenne; blood tests afterwards showed an impressive surge in blood-clot dissolving activity. Other studies have shown that Cayenne can help clear excess cholesterol from the body. The surge was short-lived – but in a comparison study, Thais with a Cayenne habit were more immune to clotting problems than Americans living in Thailand but eating it only occasionally.

N.B. Cayenne is not for everyone; if you are a hot-blooded person, or suffering from any kind of inflammatory condition, eat it sparingly or not at all.

Stress is a common cause of heart and circulatory problems, particularly high blood pressure. Even cholesterol levels – popularly associated with bingeing on eggs and cream – can be affected by stress. (US biochemist Jeffrey Bland tells of a patient from whom he had just taken a blood sample to measure her cholesterol level. On leaving his surgery, she crashed her car into a tree, and returned much shaken to the surgery. Bland took another blood sample, and was startled to find her cholesterol levels significantly higher than before.) If stress and fraying nerves could explain your case of high blood pressure, consult The Nervous System.

Cholesterol is an essential component of our body tissues; it is supplied in our diet in the form of animal proteins such as milk, eggs, butter and meat. This yellow fat was once viewed as the villain of the heart-disease story – fearful stuff, to be banished from the diet, and anxiously monitored in the body. If necessary, cholesterol-reducing drugs were prescribed, to be taken for a lifetime. The anti-cholesterol campaign is slowing down now, but there is no doubt that very high levels in your blood are bad news, and that reckless indulgence in such foods is unwise.

As well as moderating saturated fat intake, eat plenty of fibre, in the form of wholegrain cereals and vegetables; get plenty of vitamin C in your diet – fresh fruits, salads and green vegetables. Eat fresh young **Dandelion** leaves too; this wonderful blood-building plant is an excellent tonic for the circulatory system.

Limeflower is exciting more and more interest in herbal circles, for its usefulness in treating the high blood pressure that results from arteriosclerosis and stress. Culpeper noted, incidentally, that Lime flowers were 'a good cephalic and nervine, excellent for apoplexy . . . vertigo and palpitations of the heart'.

Yarrow is prescribed by herbalists for high blood pressure and the threat of blood clotting, or thrombosis. Its dilating effect on peripheral circulation makes it helpful for varicose veins and piles too. An infusion made by pouring a cupful of boiling water over 1–2 tsps of the dried herb, and steeping 10–15 minutes, can be drunk regularly, over long periods of time. Infusion of Yarrow can also be used as a lotion for compresses on painful varicose veins.

Rosemary – a cheery herb – is a grand tonic to the whole system, and helps normalize low blood pressure. It can also counter the fatigue and depression that often accompany low blood pressure. You can take Rosemary in the form of an infusion, 25g/1oz to a litre/1¾ pints of boiling water. You can add 3-4 drops of essential oil of Rosemary to a mood-lifting bath. Or you can make your own Rosemary wine: add 50g/2oz of the fresh plant to a litre/1¾ pints of good red wine; enjoy a small glassful after dinner.

Varicose veins develop when the pumping action of the calf muscles is not enough to keep the blood flowing steadily back up through the veins of the legs and thighs. The blood flow slows and the valves stop working; pooling blood stretches the veins to produce those wriggly knots of blue. Further down the line comes discomfort, cramps, varicose eczema and eventually varicose ulcers, which are slow to heal.

Varicose veins are an unrewarding malady for home doctoring in this respect: if you persevere you do not see any change – they simply do not get worse. So whatever of the following treatments you decide on, make it a habit and stick to it; doing it occasionally, or for a week or so, is a waste of effort.

There is plenty you can do about varicose veins, though. Check your diet; walk up stairs; put your feet up when you have a chance. And if you cannot resist that long, hot bath – disastrous for varicose veins, alas – at least give your legs a good cold splash and a friction with astringent **Witch-Hazel** afterwards. Do this last thing every night, too; keep a bottle in the fridge.

The bioflavonoid rutin is particularly useful; found in the leaves of **Buckwheat**, it strengthens fragile capillaries, and helps lower high blood pressure at the same time. You can take it in the form of an infusion, but as it needs to be drunk regularly, buy it in tablet form, and take some every morning. **Bee Pollen** sup-

plies rutin as well as the antioxidant vitamins C and E.

The essential oil of **Cypress** has a powerful astringent effect on veins; add a few drops to a bland cream or oil, and 2 or 3 nights a week, use some to give your legs a gentle upward stroking (*not* a massage – bad for varicose veins).

If varicose veins are already uncomfortable, bathe them with a mixture of Witch-Hazel and a strong infusion of **Marigold**. (Keep this in the fridge for no longer than a week, then make a fresh supply.) Swab on morning and evening, and at night; leave compresses on your legs, kept in place with a lint bandage. Alternatively, stroke Marigold ointment upwards over the veins. Or use a tincture of Marigold, which will tone vein walls as well as easing discomfort. Astringent **Agrimony** will help tighten slack vein-walls. Among other herbs that act to improve peripheral circulation are **Cayenne** and **Ginger**.

Varicose ulcers develop because of slowed circulation in the area, often following quite minor injuries; they can be very resistant to treatment. In the philosophy of natural medicine, no abscess or ulcer should be healed or closed up too quickly: so it makes sense to check the efficiency of your eliminative organs (see Cleansing, p.87). Take a course of a good blood-cleansing tea while you are treating the ulcer – **Burdock** or **Dandelion**.

A **Cabbage** leaf poultice can clear up varicose ulcers completely; distinguished French doctors and herbalists swear by it. The Cabbage has a unique and extraordinary ability to draw out toxins, as you will discover if you persevere. Use the dark green crinkly kind, fresh – and if possible, organically grown.

The following technique has worked for thousands of patients, according to Dr Valnet. Pick off a number of leaves and wash them well. Snip out the thick central ribs and other very prominent ones, then crush the leaves with a rolling pin until the juice just starts to appear here and there. If the ulcer is very sore, soak the leaves in **Olive** oil for an hour or so first. Then place 3 or 4 thicknesses of leaf over the ulcer; use a crepe bandage to keep in place. This should be wrapped firmly but not tightly around the limb to an inch or so above and below the ulcer. Leave on night and morning for an hour to begin with; then gradually increase the time until you are leaving it on overnight. The compress may be painful at first, as tissues start to react, but it will soon calm and the pain will go. The used leaves may be thick with serous matter drawn out from the ulcer; if so use smaller leaves and overlap them like the tiles of a roof, so that any pus is not trapped in contact with the ulcer.

Comfrey is a great herbal healer, with an extraordinary ability to regenerate damaged tissue. Get supplies of it in both whole root and powdered form. Make a small decoction by simmering a little of the root in ½ cupful of water for 10-15 minutes. Then use this to make a paste with the powdered herb; smear it thickly over a piece of lint or gauze and apply to the ulcer; bandage into place. Leave on overnight. Herbalist Anne McIntyre suggests alternating the Comfrey poultice with honey, which is wonderful for clearing out ulcers. Instead of moistening the powder with a decoction of more Comfrey, you can use other healing herbs: a strong infusion of either **Marigold, Chamomile, Rosemary, Sage** or **Thyme** can also be used as they are all good disinfectants.

Make a decoction of **Horsetail** – 50-100g/2-4oz of the fresh plant, 20g/under 1oz of the dried – simmered in a litre/1¾ pints of water for 30 minutes: use cooled and strained as compresses, or a wash. Horsetail, with its high silicon content, helps prevent scarring and rebuilds connective tissue.

Agrimony is another astringent herb that can help with ulcers. French herbalists boil 50g/2oz of the dried plant in a litre/1¾ pints of red wine for 5 minutes, then take it off the heat and let it infuse for 3 days. Strain, bottle, and use in compresses on the ulcers. The tannins in the wine reinforce the astringent action. Any old plonk will do for this.

Piles can be excruciating agony. For emergency treatment, soak a big pad of cotton-wool in ice-cold **Witch-Hazel**, and apply it. Witch-Hazel is the classic remedy – there is nothing better. You can enhance its effectiveness by steeping some Marigold flowers in Witch-Hazel for a day or two. They should then be strained before using the liquid as specified above.

There are numerous other country remedies for this complaint. What else could **Pilewort** be good for? Otherwise known as the Lesser Celandine, astringent Pilewort is usually applied in the form of an ointment, which any chemist used to stock. Nowadays they do not, but it is very easy to make. Here is the formula for *Unguentum Ficariae BPC* from the 1911 British Pharmaceutical Codex: 350g/4oz Pilewort herb cut up into pieces. Add it to 3 times its weight of melted lard, and allow it to digest at 38°C (body temperature) for 24 hours in an

---

FOR PILES
Take a pint of Elderberys and halfe a pint of linseed oyle boile these till they come to a salve. Keep it for your use and when you use it spread it on a cloth.

Physicall Receipts
(Elizabeth Jacob, 1654)

---

airing cupboard, next to a boiler or in an oven with the pilot light on; then strain, press and add sufficient lard to produce the required weight.

Boiled till they were soft with a little **Linseed** oil, the green leaves of the **Elder** tree were another country remedy for piles, so often recorded and recopied that it must have been efficacious. Until well into this century, chemists sold a Green Elder ointment, made from 3 parts of the green leaves to 4 of lard and 2 of suet, heated together till the leaves lost their colour; then strained through a linen cloth and cooled. This cooling, soothing and softening ointment was used for wounds and bruises and chilblains too.

The leaves should be picked within 3-4 days of their first unfolding, when they are only 1-2 inches long.

Elderberries seem to have been used in much the same way.

Herbalist Ann Warren-Davis once remarked to me that a number of her patients who were sensitive to dairy products often complained of piles too. When a possible connection was suggested, several of them were able to confirm it from their own experience. Cheese – particularly blue vein – could aggravate the condition almost overnight in some cases. Could this be your problem? Worth a little experimentation to find out.

When a pharmaceutical company surveyed a number of British women recently, they found that an incredible 1 in 12 suffered from chilblains – some of them so severely that halfway through winter their shoes no longer fitted, and walking was agony. Chilblains are a mild form of frostbite, caused by severe restriction of the small blood vessels just under the skin;

fingers and toes turn purply-red, become numbed, then itch agonizingly as circulation returns.

I remember one of my sisters suffering mild chilblains as a child one winter; she was despatched into the garden to run around barefoot in the snow for 5 minutes, while we all watched giggling. This country cure was completely effective: chilblains occur because of poor circulation (see the suggestions for varicose veins, and circulation generally, above).

If you develop chilblains when there is no snow, resist the temptation to stick your poor feet on a radiator or in front of the fire to thaw them out. Instead, try alternating footbaths of hot and cold water, finishing with cold, and a brisk rub. If you are a chilly person anyway, you need more exercise outdoors in winter, not less – as long as you are well wrapped up. 'Warm the person, not the room,' Swedish natural healer Are Waerland used to say.

Meanwhile, there are lots of effective remedies for those chilblains, featuring herbs which kickstart the circulation locally or soothe the inflammation and irritation. Squeeze a vitamin E capsule on to them. Paint them with tincture, or oil, of **Cayenne**. Apply grated fresh **Horseradish** root, bandaged into place. Paint them with fresh **Lemon** or **Garlic** or **Onion** juice. Or try tincture of **Benzoin**; ask for this at your local chemist under the delightful name Friar's Balsam.

Dr Valnet suggests **Celery** as a remedy for chilblains; numbers of people have confirmed to him its efficacy. Take 250g/10oz of either the Celery stalks, or the peelings of the lumpy knobbly root – greengrocers sell it as **Celeriac**. Simmer them in a litre/1¾ pints of water for an hour, then give yourself a footbath, as hot as you can bear it, 3 times a day.

THE DIGESTIVE SYSTEM

Nausea, gas, belching, farting, heartburn, constipation, stomach-cramps, griping, 'the runs', wind . . . what a lowly set of problems. The remedy is as lowly as the problem – kitchen medicine. The kitchen is usually where the problem starts, and it is the best place to go for the remedy.

Digestive problems can have a number of causes. Stress can be a major factor; some people really take it out on their stomachs – and the price of success is often an ulcer. Achievers like this are usually tense, rapid eaters too, which does not help. If stress is giving you ulcers, look at the chapter on the Nervous System, p.108; there is little point in clearing up the ulcer if the stress persists.

You do not need to be a tycoon to eat badly, however. Most of us eat too much, too fast, too often, too richly. Paradoxically, we do not *enjoy* our food enough: the good things of the earth are meant to be delicious. Foodies are much less likely to suffer from indigestion than the rest of us; Slow Food is healthy food.

We need to learn to eat only when we are hungry, with appetite, taking our time over it, and enjoying every mouthful. Then we will seldom, if ever, need any of the homely, harmless remedies in the following pages.

Carrots have been called the great friend of the intestines; they calm and heal the irritated gut wall, and sort out both diarrhoea and constipation. Grate a Carrot into every salad you make, add Carrots to soups; a thin purée is a country remedy for diarrhoea.

Or try a handful of sun-dried **Onion** skins simmered for 10 minutes in 1 litre/1¾ pints of water. Drink 2 or 3 wineglassfuls a day. Buy organically grown Onions, or grow your own

– pesticide-free.

Extra-virgin **Olive** oil, so richly enjoyable, is the oil your liver prefers too. In Mediterranean folk medicine, a spoonful taken first thing in the morning is good for most kinds of stomach upset, stressed liver, or constipation. If you find the taste too rich, add a teaspoon of **Lemon** juice. Repeat every morning till the problem has cleared.

N.B. Some people have an impaired ability to absorb fats; if the Olive oil treatment fails to produce a result within 2-3 days, stop it.

An Ayurvedic remedy for diarrhoea is as follows. Grate a teaspoon of fresh **Ginger** root into a cup; fill it with half-and-half plain, live yogurt and water; grate in a little **Nutmeg**.

Barley Water is not only nourishing, it is a tonic to the liver, and is helpful in controlling diarrhoea. To make it, put 100g/4oz of pot Barley in a pan, just cover with water and bring to the boil. Strain, discarding the water and put back in the pan. Add a litre/1¾ pints of water, and the peel of one well-scrubbed **Lemon**. Bring to the boil, and simmer gently until the Barley is soft. Add more water from time to time. Then strain, and stir in 2tbsp of honey.

Umeboshi plums are the extremely sour, sun-dried and salt-pickled plums of the Japanese Ume tree. The longer they are left in brine, the more valuable they are medicinally. They are a Macrobiotic remedy for acute conditions such as diarrhoea, hangovers, dysentery or food poisoning; or for chronic conditions due to overload of acid wastes in the system, such as fatigue, constipation or morning sickness. Umeboshi are spectacularly high in alkalizing salts; it has been calculated that 10g can neutralize the acid wastes from eating 100g/4oz of sugar. Umeboshi plums can be cooked with rice, chewed as they are or soaked in a cupful of hot Bancha tea. Then drink the tea and eat the plum. You can buy both plums and Bancha tea at good health-food shops.

A German physician, Dr Kutroff, cured many cases of dysentery, often severe, with **Apples**: he gave his patients 1½ kilos – about 3½ lbs – of grated raw Apples daily. Patients were also allowed to chew raw Apples. The Apples should be grated on a plastic grater, and eaten immediately, 6 times a day. Nothing else should be eaten. The Apples, with their high pectin content, soak up toxins in the intestine; freshly pressed Apple juice has also been found to have formidable bactericidal powers. Try this for cases of mild food poisoning or diarrhoea; more severe cases could be dysentery, however, and should always be referred to a doctor.

When bitter herbs such as **Tansy, Wormwood** or **Gentian** come in contact with the bitter receptors in the mouth they trigger secretion from the stomach wall of the hormone gastrin, which sharpens appetite and boosts the output of the digestive juices and of bile. Wormwood and Gentian are both ingredients of popular *aperitifs*; the French make Gentian wine, to be sipped before meals, and Italians like to accompany their after-dinner coffee – itself quite bitter – with an *Amaro*. In the Middle Ages Tansy was eaten in the form of little cakes at the end of Lent – perhaps in preparation for the great Easter blow-out. Tansy leaves or a little of the juice was also added to omelettes, sauces and salads. **N.B.** Pregnant women should avoid Tansy. And if you are already suffering from acid stomach, or an ulcer, obviously avoid bitters. But as an occasional tonic for a lazy digestion, try **Dandelion** root coffee after dinner; Dandelions are a wonderful tonic for your liver too.

Surprisingly, **Chamomile** flowers are another bitter herb; but if you drink Chamomile tea as a *digestif*, do not sweeten it.
Another popular digestive drink, served to non-coffee drinkers in Italy, is a *canarino*. A long curl of very finely pared **Lemon** peel is infused in a cup of boiling water for a few minutes. The water turns a beautiful bright yellow, and is drunk unsweetened. Lemons are a useful stimulant to the liver. **N.B.** Use unwaxed Lemons.

Hops are yet another bitter herb. This is an old recipe for Hop Bitters, quoted by Mrs Grieve in *A Modern Herbal*. Take 12g/½oz Hops, 25g/1oz **Angelica** herb, and 25g/1oz **Holy Thistle**. Pour 1¾ litres/3 pints of boiling water on them and strain when cold. A wineglassful may be taken 4 times a day.
When certain foods ferment, the *lactobacillus acidophilus* is at work to produce lactic acid. Foods rich in lactic acid keep the digestive tract sweet by hindering the multiplication of the micro-organisms responsible for putrefaction in the gut. Fermented foods are used in almost every culture as a supreme health-food, and a remedy for digestive upsets of every kind: the *kefir* of Russia and the *koumiss* of the Crimea; the fermented soya relishes and the umeboshi plums of Japan; the whey of Switzerland; the sauerkraut of Germany; the pickled gherkins and cucumbers of northern Europe; the buttermilk of North American frontier medicine. Cottage cheese is also a lactic acid food. Sauerkraut is particularly valuable for digestive upsets and diarrhoea, since Cabbage is a powerful anti-putrefactive and a friend to the digestive tract. The best sauerkraut is made

without chemicals, and sold in health-food stores or Jewish delicatessens. Do not rinse it; serve it as it is, with a spoonful of live yogurt.

Many health-food shops sell the juice pressed from sauerkraut, found in research by Professor Dr Kemkes at the Institute of Hygiene of the University of Giessen to be an excellent treatment for chronic constipation, because of its high lactic acid content.

The **Cabbage**-leaf treatment for diarrhoea, dysentery or a painfully congested liver can be carried out even if you are already receiving medical treatment; it will greatly speed up recovery. Wash big, fresh green Cabbage leaves, snip out the thick ribs, flatten with an iron or a rolling-pin, and put 3 or 4 layers of them over the painful area; cover with a piece of linen and bind firmly into place with a crepe bandage. Leave on for 4 hours, or overnight. The power of the Cabbage leaf to draw out toxins from deep inside tissue is acknowledged by many

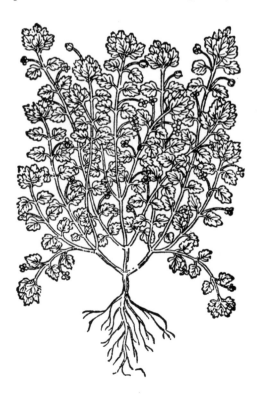

In 1747, Mrs Howard had a Niece, naturally of a ruddy Complection, and of a sound Constitution, but the Mother of it having indulged the Girl (almost six Years old) in drinking Tea every Morning, and sometimes in the Afternoon, she fell into the Jaundice, but was cured by Mrs Howard, *who only gave her a Spoonful of Chickweed-juice fasting, and another Spoonful at four of the Clock in the Afternoon in a little Ale; but it would not be amiss if a little Saffron was mixt with the Juice. This was continued till perfectly cured, and she tells me that this has done, when all other Remedies have failed. The Saffron by tincturing the Juice makes it excellent. N.B. The Juice of Chickweed has cured several grown Persons about Market-street in Hertfordshire.*

The Country Housewife's
Family Companion
(W. Ellis, 1750)

French doctors (see The Circulatory System). For chronic diarrhoea: eat raw young, globe **Artichokes** in salad.

For painful indigestion after meals, Danièle Ryman suggests chewing a few **Caraway** seeds slowly, drinking a glass of warm water, and breathing deeply for 10 minutes.

Better still, put a teaspoon of Caraway seeds in a pan, cover with water, bring to the boil and simmer for 10 minutes. Cool a little and sip slowly before meals.

Chickweed is soothing and healing to the whole digestive tract, as well as being a wonderful food. Wash it and eat it chopped into a salad; it needs something sharp and biting with it, to offset its rather insipid taste.

Another remedy for diarrhoea is as follows: a handful of brown **Rice** – well washed – in 250ml/8floz of water. Boil till the liquid is reduced by half, then take a soupspoon every 30 minutes. Use organically-grown rice.

Cold green **Tea** is a folk remedy for mild diarrhoea or any kind of irritation of the gut wall, taken without milk or sugar. The tannins help check inflammation and infection. Choose a good tea such as Gunpowder. Many herbs have this kind of astringent action – **Tormentil, Bistort, Goldenseal** and **Agrimony** among them.

Many health problems are due to an excess of acid wastes in the system, and health farms and sanatoria put their patients on an Alkaline Broth regime, to counter this acidity. The US food guru of the 1960s, Gayelord Hauser, reinvented it as Eliminative Broth, made with **Carrots, Celery, Spinach, Tomatoes** and **Parsley. Leeks** and **Courgettes** are also very

alkalizing. One of the essential ingredients, **Celery**, is famous as a cure for hyperacidity problems such as gout, arthritis, rheumatism or a tendency to stone; it is also a fine tonic to the kidneys. Drink a small glass of Celery juice, freshly pressed, or a good bottled one before midday and evening meals.

Raw **Potato** juice is a famous old remedy for severe gastric problems, including ulcers. In a study carried out by doctors, 90 per cent of patients said they felt better after just 2 days of the cure; after 5-10 days, they had no more trouble. Use organically-grown potatoes, peeled, and be careful to avoid those with any green bits – indicating the presence of a poisonous alkaloid. The dose is 50ml/1¾floz before meals, 3 times a day. It has to be said that raw Potato juice is not very nice; you can add a spoonful of **Lemon** juice, or tip it into a tepid soup. Alternatively, you can take freshly-pressed **Cabbage** juice instead, or **Carrot** juice.

JOINTS AND MUSCLES

All foods 'burned' – in other words, digested – in our bodies leave an 'ash' that is either acid, neutral, or alkaline. The pH, or acid-alkaline balance of our blood plasma must remain at a steady 7.35-7.45; an excess either way tips us into crisis, even death. To preserve this vital balance, acids are neutralized in our bodies by the alkaline salts – sodium, potassium, calcium, magnesium and others – found in fruit and vegetables.

If there is a healthy balance in our diet between alkaline and acid foods – estimated at a ratio of 4:1 – then we enjoy excellent health. Imbalance spells trouble; much the most common imbalance is excess acidity, when our

alkaline reserves are grossly depleted. Unneutralized acid wastes from our diet join cell debris and other metabolic wastes produced by normal metabolic processes. Stress and long spells of overwork produce further acid wastes, all of which pile up in body tissues. In Nature Cure, the resulting condition is called toxaemia; it is considered responsible for many health problems, and for degenerative diseases such as arthritis, rheumatism and gout.

The first concern of the herbalist or Natural Medicine practitioner treating such disease is to ensure that wastes are efficiently and speedily eliminated, and the system restored to a healthy balance (see Cleansing, p.89).

A good balanced diet is vital: many cases clear up quickly when bad eating habits are corrected. Particularly to be avoided: processed foods containing artificial sweeteners. See 'What is Healthy Eating?' p. 22.

Stress can be a major factor in joint problems; if this could be the case for you, see The Nervous System, p.108.

The professional herbalist can call on many herbs which will help treat the root causes of rheumatic and joint problems, as well as easing the aches and pains of the patients or helping deal with stress or anxiety conditions. If you have a competent practitioner within your reach, he or she will sort out just which herbs will be particularly beneficial for your case. Among these might be the so-called Alteratives — herbs which improve general metabolism, usually by cleansing the blood or boosting elimination; good examples are **Celery** seed or **Guaiacum**. There are also anti-inflammatories, such as **Meadowsweet**, and diuretics such as **Dandelion**, herbs which help cleanse wastes. There are circulatory stimulants, such as **Prickly Ash**, which will not only get things moving generally, but can also be applied topically to ease pain.

Many herbs carry out almost all these functions simultaneously; the suggestions below are all for mild, safe herbs which can be — indeed, need to be — taken for weeks at a time. None of the suggested herbs is likely to be of any use unless taken regularly over at least 3 weeks; herbal medicine is sure but slow, particularly in the case of chronic conditions which may have been developing over years.

Joint problems can be yet another manifestation of food intolerance. The Hay Diet is often successful at clearing up such conditions, even after months or years of suffering. Briefly, this regime consists of avoiding the combination of concentrated starches — such as bread, potatoes or rice — and concentrated proteins — such as steak, scampi and cheese — at the same meal. See *Food Combining for Health* by Doris Grant and Jean Joice (Thorsons) and *The Superfoods Diet Book* by Michael van Straten and Barbara Griggs (Dorling Kindersley), for further details.

Dr Alfred Vogel, whose book *The Nature Doctor* has sold in huge quantities all over Europe, suggests a simple if drastic cure for cases for rheumatism, arthritis and gout. Cut out completely any food with excess acidity, and replace it with foods that are high in alkalinity. 'In other words the patient must go without meat, fish, eggs and cheese.'

Instead, he proposes a big breakfast of muesli made with plenty of **fruit, honey** and **Almonds**; lunch or supper should be built round **Potatoes, Millet**, brown **Rice** or **Buckwheat**, eaten with plenty of fresh vegetables, salads, and cottage cheese. Drink fresh mixed vegetable juices — particularly **Carrot, White Cabbage** and **Kale** — instead of wine, and try to have a one-day fast, drinking nothing but vegetable juices or a good bottled spring water such as Evian, once or twice a week.

As a specific remedy for arthritis, Dr Vogel recommends **Potato** juice — from at least one potato daily — sipped slowly fasting in the morning. Use organically grown potatoes. If you find the taste horrible, add it to warm water or soup. If you do not have a juicer, scrub a medium Potato, slice it thinly into a food processor and process for a minute or so. Add a cupful of water and process until the Potato is a heavy pulp. Turn out into a mug. Add a squeeze of Lemon juice, let it stand for 10 minutes, then strain and drink. Or you can buy an excellent, Swiss-made Potato juice, in most health-food shops.

Eat lots of **Celery**, and drink a daily half-glass of Celery juice for a three-week cure when your joints are particularly painful. In Japan, rheumatic patients are put on a Celery-only cure for a week or two at a time.

A similar powder, called *Pulvis Apii Compositum*, is still sold in Italian pharmacies.

N.B. Use with caution – pregnant women should avoid it altogether.

For those who are so tormented with gout that even their mouth is deformed and twisted and their limbs tremble and they are tense and contracted in their limbs: let them reduce to powder the seeds of Celery and add to them a third part of Rue, and a quantity of Nutmeg slightly smaller than the powdered Rue, and a quantity of Cloves in a smaller quantity than the Nutmeg, and Saxifrage in a smaller quantity than the Cloves. And let him reduce all these herbs to powder and let them eat this powder either fasting or after meals, and the gout will go away because this is the best treatment for gout.

St Hildegarde of Bingen
(Twelfth Century)

Dandelions are another Super Cleanser for aching joints and muscles – as well as an enjoyable food.

Globe Artichokes promote the elimination of bile and cholesterol, lowering levels of urea and uric acid in the blood; good news for the rheumatic and gouty.

The oils of fatty fish such as salmon and sardines can help shut down the inflammatory process that make arthritis agony. The omega-3 fatty acids in these fish-oils damp down production in the body of chemicals called B4 leukotrienes, which trigger inflammation.

Country people with rheumatic knees used to slip a **Cabbage** leaf over the joint inside their stockings. The Cabbage is friend to the gouty and rheumatic too; applied locally, it can give great relief. Cabbage compresses (for details see p.96) can be applied to aching joints, covered with a wool bandage, and left on for a few hours or overnight. Or make hot poultices of Cabbage cooked in wine, and drink a small glass or two of fresh Cabbage juice daily, unless you find it too windy for comfort.

Comfrey tea is an old-fashioned remedy for gout in the feet. Make a strong infusion of the leaves, using 3-4 litres (6 pints or so) of water, let it cool a little, then sit with both feet in it for 15-20 minutes.

Strawberries were once forbidden fruit for the gouty; Linnaeus thought otherwise. In fact both Strawberries and **Raspberries** are wonderful cleansers, as are **Cherries**, which specifically help clear uric acid from the system; in the Cherry season, try a cleansing two-day mono-fast on Cherries – no great hardship! Choose the dark red ones, and eat them when they are ripe.

In the spring-time, eat fresh young **Nettle**-tops once a week. Nettles are rich in alkaloids that help neutralize uric acids. Nettle tea can be drunk at any time of the year, made from the dried leaves (see p.47).

Austrian herbalist Maria Treben suggests a Nettle bath; soak a bucketful of fresh stinging Nettles or 200g/8oz of dried Nettles in cold water for 12 hours. Then gently heat up the infusion, strain, and pour it into your bath.

An Italian country remedy for gout and rheumatism: add 80g/just over 3oz of dried **Elderflowers** to a litre/1¾ pints of good red wine vinegar. Let them macerate in the sun or a warm place for 8-10 days; then strain and take a couple of dessertspoonfuls a day.

Lignum vitae or **Guaiacum** was first imported from the Spanish West Indies in the early sixteenth century as a miracle-cure for the epidemic of a 'new' disease, syphilis, which was ravaging Europe – rather as Aids does today. Now it is considered specific for painful rheumatic conditions, which it helps by boosting circulation, raising a mild perspiration, and by its diuretic action. Take a teaspoon of the wood chips in a cup of water; bring to the boil and simmer for 15-20 minutes. Drink 3 times daily.

A person said that Nettle-tea drunk half a pint in a morning fasting, if continued long enough, will cure any rheumatism.

The Country Housewife's Family
Companion
(W. Ellis, 1750)

------○------

Prickly Ash is the perfect remedy for those suffering from chronic rheumatism, arthritis and other joint problems, who are also chilly, with weak digestions. It is a powerfully stimulating and energizing herb, a warming pain reliever. Famous US herbalist Dr John Christopher combines it with other useful anti-rheumatics in this formula: 12g/½oz Prickly Ash bark; 12g/½oz Buckbean or Bogbean; 12g/½oz Guaiacum chips; ½tsp Cayenne powder. Boil for 15 minutes in 900ml/1½ pints of water; strain. Take a wineglassful 3-4 times daily. He also suggests adding 25g/1oz of powdered Prickly Ash bark to 100g/4oz of **Olive** oil, and rubbing it into painful joints.

The great anti-rheumatic discovery of the century has been **Devil's Claw**, from South-West Africa, used by Namibian tribesmen for centuries. It was brought to Western attention

by a German farmer who had settled locally, was impressed by its reputation, and sent samples back to Germany for clinical research. Numerous studies have now been carried out in Germany and in France; they have established beyond doubt that Devil's Claw can be extremely effective for both rheumatoid and osteo-arthritis, countering pain, swelling and stiffness. It appears to act both as detoxifier and stimulant.

Devil's Claw does not work for everyone; but it is worth giving it a month's trial to see if it will solve your problems. In tea form the dose is ½-1tsp of the powdered root, simmered in a cupful of water for 10-15 minutes, taken 3 times a day. Or you can take it in tablet form. Devil's Claw also appears to boost elimination of uric acid and excessive cholesterol; its only unwanted side-effect seems to be that it is laxative in some people.

N.B. Devil's Claw has been known to lower the diabetic's need for insulin; if you are diabetic, discuss this with your doctor.

British herbalists value the common **Chickweed** for their rheumatic patients. 'It should be thought of,' says Nalda Gosling, 'when pains are sharp and darting in any part of the body. It helps rheumatoid arthritis in different parts of the body; stiffness of joints; pains in shoulders and arms and calves of legs. It also aids digestion. (Deficiency in the digestive enzymes, as well as stress, can be one of the contributing factors in the development of rheumatism).' The dose she suggests is this: 38g/1½oz of the dried herb, or 50g/2oz of the fresh in 900ml/1½ pints of water boiled down to 1 pint. Strain and take ½ a teacupful every 2 or 3 hours.

Modern French trials of **Canadian Fleabane** have lent truth to what Culpeper wrote of 'Flea Wort' centuries ago, 'It helps all inflammation in any part of the body, and the pains that come thereby, as . . . the pains of the gout and the sciatica.' This rather drab-looking tall weed with the insignificant white flowers has grey seeds which looked just like fleas, thought Culpeper.

Fleabane is today highly valued as a diuretic, eliminator of uric acid, and anti-inflammatory by French phytotherapists treating gout and rheumatism. Put a dessertspoon of the whole plant, cut up, in a cupful of water; bring to the boil, simmer for 2 minutes, then infuse for 10. Take 3 cups a day, between meals.

The fruit and leaves of the **Blackcurrant** are equally helpful for those suffering from rheumatism and arthritis. Both help counter acidity, are diuretic, and contain plenty of vitamin C in a particularly stable form. If you have a Blackcurrant bush of your own, harvest and dry the leaves carefully; they are a treasury of medicine. See Tea-Time, p.47, for a Blackcurrant tea recipe. Take 3-4 cupfuls of tea a day.

Dr Henri Leclerc, one of France's most revered phyotherapists, suggested this formula for chronic rheumatism and gout: 50g/2oz dried Blackcurrant leaves; 25g/1oz each of dried Ash leaves, and the dried flowering tops of Meadowsweet. Add a tablespoonful of this mixture to a cup of boiling water and infuse for 10 minutes. Drink 3 times a day between meals.

Palaiseul suggests an alternative. Add about 20 fresh Blackcurrant leaves to 1 litre/1¾ pints of good white wine; let them macerate for 10-15 days. Then strain and add a drop or two of *cassis*; drink a wineglassful before dinner.

Or drink plain unsweetened Blackcurrant juice, home-made if possible; commercial juices are usually heavily sweetened. If you do not have a juicer, buy the fresh or frozen fruit and eat it puréed.

. . . I was consulted by a market gardener condemned to inaction and considerable pain by a sacro-iliac arthritis. Since added to these woes was the irritation of seeing his land overrun by the Fleabane which ran riot there, I persuaded him to make use of this evil weed to combat his own painful and obstinate affliction. He had a strong decoction made – 150g to a litre of water – of which he drank 3 glasses every morning. This treatment produced the happiest results; so much so that the patient who formerly rained curses on the intrusive weed was now to be seen gazing at it . . . with a mixture of gratitude and resentment. . . .

Precis de Phytotherapie
(Henri Leclerc)

Meadowsweet contains a chemical called salicylic acid, first isolated in the early nineteenth century by an Italian pharmacologist. From this, in 1899, acetylsalicylic acid – much less irritating to the stomach – was derived and named after Meadowsweet, or *Spiraea ulmaria*. Meadowsweet is a powerful eliminator of uric acid; because of these diuretic properties it helps counter the pain of aching, arthritic joints or gout.

Make an infusion by adding 40-50g/2oz of the dried flowering tops to a litre/1¾ pints of water, brought to about 90° – not boiling point – and infused covered for 10 minutes. Drink 3-4 cupfuls a day, between meals. For the treatment to be effective, follow it for 3 weeks. Hot compresses of the infusion can help relieve pain locally, too; or use the discarded flowers.

Swollen joints may be soothed, and much toxic waste eliminated, with the help of an infusion of **Ash** leaves; these are both laxative and diuretic, as well as anti-inflammatory. Add a handful to a litre/1¾ pints of boiling water, and infused for 10 minutes. Take a wineglassful 3 times a day. The same infusion can be used as a hot compress on the joints.

Compresses of **Cider** vinegar – as hot as can be borne without blistering – also help aching joints. Soak a cloth in the hot vinegar and renew as often as it cools.

Ginger up your circulation to help arthritic pains in the joints or strained and aching muscles. Take 1-2 inches of fresh Ginger root; grate or crush it into 200ml/7floz of warming Sesame oil, and leave overnight. Next morning, press the oil through a cloth, and use to massage painful joints or muscles.

I have found that Roses allay rheumatic pain. A handful of petals thrown into the bath will do wonders. The same discovery has been made by someone I know, a wealthy industrialist who shares my passion for flowers. He amused himself by throwing handfuls of rose petals from his garden into his bath from time to time, and observed that he was no longer bothered by rheumatic aches. One day he mentioned the matter to me and I assured him that this was the effect of his roses.

Maurice Messegue's Way
to Natural Health and Beauty

'Our family has been using grated Ginger baths for years,' says herbalist Dian Dincin Buchman, who votes Ginger one of her favourite herbs. 'Ginger baths are great for circulation, and will decrease muscle soreness and muscle stiffness.' It is good for inflamed and aching joints, too. Add a couple of teaspoons of powdered Ginger, or slice an inch or so of

the root, into a litre/1¾ pints of water; simmer till it turns yellow, then pour it into your bath. Wrap up warmly when you get out of the bath and go to bed: but first, very gently, exercise those stiff joints for a couple of minutes.

Use hot Ginger tea as a compress, too – it will have excellent results.

Ginger scored full marks in a small trial carried out in 1988 with 7 people suffering from rheumatoid arthritis. They were asked to take a daily dose of either fresh or powdered Ginger. All 7 reported real improvement in their condition, with less pain and swelling, more mobility in the joints, and less stiffness on waking.

Aromatherapy comes to the rescue in rheumatic problems, with a number of oils which help soothe away aches and pains, and reduce swelling and stiffness.

Lavender should be the first choice for its calming, analgesic qualities: in a massage oil it helps relax the body, ease tensed muscles. Other oils to consider are fresh-scented **Pine** which has a stimulating effect on the circulation; **Juniper**, strengthening and detoxifying; **Roman Chamomile**, an excellent anti-

---

How a Higler cured himself of a Fit of the Gout. – I am informed that one Mr. Gould, a Higler, being seized on a Journey with a Gout in his Foot, so that he could not walk, stopt at Busby near Watford, and poured some Spirit of Lavender into his Shoe, and by the Time he rode Fourteen miles to London, he was thoroughly cured.

The Country Housewife's
Family Companion
(W. Ellis, 1750)

inflammatory. **Rosemary** and strong-smelling **Eucalyptus** are both useful in massage oils to soothe stiff painful joints. **Black Pepper, Marjoram** and **Ginger** help relieve pain by their local warming and circulation-boosting qualities. Aromatherapist Shirley Price suggests this calming, anti-inflammatory mix: 5 drops each of Juniper Berry, Eucalyptus, Roman Chamomile and Lavender, in 60ml/ 2floz of carrier oil.

To make the mix – or any of these oils – even more effective, add them to **St John's** **Wort** oil. Many herbal suppliers stock this, but if it grows in your or a friend's garden, it is easy to make your own. Fill a wide-mouthed jar with the freshly-picked, just-opened flowers, giving them a good shake first to free them of dust or insects. Then fill the jar up to the top with Olive oil, close it up tightly, and stand on a sunny window-sill for 4–6 weeks until the oil has turned a dramatic deep red. Strain out the oil, squeezing out the last drops from the flowers, and rebottle. The oil on its own is useful for nerve or muscle pain.

THE NERVOUS SYSTEM

Stress, fatigue, nervous exhaustion, clinical depression and anxiety, are late twentieth-century plagues, epidemic in our hustling, frantic times. Bombarded with bad news from the world over; assailed by noise and pollution; crowded into packed commuter trains and buses for the twice-daily slog to work; hurried over meals; and far too often racing against the clock – we live life today as a speed that would have made our ancestors of even a century ago gasp with disbelief. No wonder that fatigue and insomnia are two of the commonest problems any GP encounters. And no wonder that anti-depressants and tranquillizers are prescribed by the million.

As the landmark research of Walter Cannon and Hans Selye showed earlier this century, stress and nervous tension may originate in the mind, but they exert a massive toll physically too, draining our nervous energy and vitality. A nervous crisis, a prolonged spell of overwork, or a bout of severe depression tend to deplete their victims physically in another way; too tired to shop, cook a decent meal or eat properly, they end up snacking on tea, coffee, sandwiches and biscuits, or turn to alcohol for instant warmth and comfort.

Conversely, eating badly can affect our minds and nervous systems as well as our bodies. Fatigue, depression, confusion, loss of memory and apathy are among the earliest symptoms of severe nutritional deficiencies – particularly of the B-complex vitamins, iron, calcium or magnesium. Eating fresh foods rich in these nutrients may be a cure in itself; it will certainly help alleviate the condition.

Long-term, the cure for these stressed conditions can only be found in radical reappraisal of lifestyle and spiritual values. Meditation, relaxation, yoga, long walks in fresh country air are all good unwinding techniques, and give us a chance to step back and reflect on our lives.

There is plenty to be done on the purely physical level too. There are wonderful herbs which can strengthen, tone and nourish the nervous system. There are herbs to help you sleep, to help you relax and unwind, to counter depression or anxiety, to help you deal with stress. Unlike tranquillizers or anti-depressants, however, the side-effects of these mild, natural 'nervines' are wholly beneficial and physiologically non-addictive.

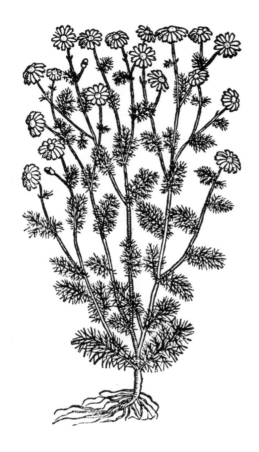

Chamomile, for instance, is a gentle sedative. **Balm** relaxes the central nervous system and helps counter tension.

The world of plants comes to our rescue with aromatherapy too, treatment with the essential oils of aromatic plants. Research is beginning to unravel the mysterious ways in which aromas can affect us mentally, emotionally or spiritually. In her book *Aromatherapy, an A-Z*, Patricia Davis cites experiments with volunteers:

who showed that such oils as Basil and Rosemary, which we associate with mental clarity, produced brain-rhythm patterns showing alertness, while the calming anti-depressants such as Jasmine, Rose and Neroli induced rhythms which showed the mind approaching a state of meditation.

Use the effective tonics, tranquillizers, relaxants and sedatives offered by the plant world; you will find simple home-remedies in the following pages. If your problems are too severe for self-treatment, consult an expert, a trained herbalist or aromatherapist (see Useful Addresses, p.158).

Millions of Brazilians today value Guarana as the indispensable, all-purpose pick-me-up and general tonic. This effect may be partially accounted for by the fact that it contains small amounts of caffeine. Research has demonstrated, however, that a high content of nutritious fats, oils and resins slows absorption of this caffeine, so there is no quick 'hit' and subsequent low, and no caffeine jitters. Instead, its action in combatting stress, fatigue, or extremes of climate is pronounced but steady.

In my own experience, Guarana is invaluable for anyone with an exceptionally high work-load, repeated sessions with the midnight oil, or extremes of climate. It allowed me to put in long days of intensive work during the high temperatures and humidity of a Roman summer; and our eldest daughter went off to do her A-levels with a daily priming of Guarana.

By the same token, save this marvellous tonic for times of real need, and take it for days, rather than weeks at a time. If caffeine is a problem for you, choose another solution.

Guarana is imported from plantations worked by the native Maues Indians (see Useful Addresses, p.158). The daily dose is two 500mg capsules of the powdered seed before breakfast: in case of need, repeat the dose mid-afternoon.

Eat lots of **Seaweed**; it supplies plenty of nerve-foods such as iron and calcium. *Hijiki* is spectacularly rich in calcium, containing 1400mg for 100g/4oz dry weight – more than 10 times as much as milk. It is also very rich in iron, with nearly 10 times more than Spinach. Over-acidity is a common cause of fatigue, and seaweeds are also highly alkalizing. Make sure that your source is a pollution-free one: try the Clearspring range.

Wood Betony was once prized as the sovereign remedy for all pains and aches in the head, and cultivated in monastery physic gardens all over Europe. As late as our own century, it was still being drunk both as a healthy substitute for tea and as preventative medicine for those disposed to nervous headaches. To make it, pour 600ml/a pint of boiling water on 25g/1oz of the dried herb, and infuse for 10 minutes. Drink a wineglassful 3 times a day. Modern herbalists prescribe it as 'an excellent remedy for all head and face pains, and for nervous troubles.' Try this tea: 25g/1oz each of Wood Betony, Rosemary herb and Peppermint. Pour 300ml/½ pint of boiling water over a quarter of this mixture, and cover closely until cool. Strain and sweeten to taste, and take 3tbsp every 2 hours until the headache is better. Then take 3tbsp 4 times a day. (Make a fresh batch daily.)

Rosemary, among its range of uses, is valued today by aromatherapists for its dynamizing effect on the entire system, a general stimulant to the nervous system, the heart, and the adrenal cortex. It is used in a number of ways to counter general debility and fatigue, mental strain and loss of memory. If you are under severe stress, drink weak Rosemary tea once or twice a day instead of tea or coffee (see Tea-Time, p.52 for how to make it).

N.B. Pregnant women or those trying to conceive should avoid Rosemary except as an occasional flavouring.

Stress, tension and anxiety do not just drain us mentally; they translate into a physical tensing or spasm of smooth muscle all over the body, to produce such nervous symptoms as 'butterflies in the stomach', an asthma attack or an overactive bowel. There are a number of herbal relaxants that help counter such neuromuscular tension. Not so much, as Simon Mills explains, 'because these remedies prevent the symptom occurring directly, although they often will, but because, by reducing the effective impact of the tensions on the body as a whole, they permit that body to marshal more of its vital resources to coping with them.' The best-known and most effective herbal relaxant is **Valerian**, which tranquilizes without sedating, and is particularly effective at treating the insomnia caused by a buzz of anxious thoughts. Valerian is non-addictive, but Mills suggests that if you still need it after a month's use, you should consult a qualified herbal practitioner.

An infusion of the fresh Valerian root does not smell particularly appealing, so herbalists often combine it with other useful relaxants. Barbara and Peter Theiss suggest this Nerve-Calming Tea: 40g/under 2oz Valerian root, 30g/1oz Hops, 15g Peppermint leaves, 15g Hibiscus flowers. Mix all together, then pour 600ml/a pint of lukewarm water over 25g/1oz of the mixture. Leave overnight, then strain in the morning, heat to drinking temperature, and put in a thermos flask. Drink it throughout the day.

Other relaxants Simon Mills suggests are **Chamomile** or **Balm**, both helpful for digestive upsets due to nerves, and **Hops** for nervous bowel syndrome. Add 25g/1oz of any of these herbs to 600ml/a pint of boiling water and steep covered for 30 minutes.

When you are so tense from fatigue and over-work that you cannot unwind, sleep, or relax, or when you are racked by nervous headache, Roman **Chamomile** will help calm and soothe your nervous system. It contains plenty of easily assimilable calcium – a real nerve-food. The teabags you see everywhere are a very low dose, though. Buy a supply of the little flower-heads loose; use 5-10 of them to a cupful of boiling water – infuse covered for 6 minutes. Drink before meals, and another cup-ful at bedtime. For sleeplessness, brew up 500ml/¾ pint of double-strength Chamomile tea and put it in a warm bedtime bath too.

Balm has a centuries-old reputation as an in-vigorating tonic to the mind and nerves. 'Balm makes a happy heart and strengthens the spirit,' said the great eleventh-century Arab physician Avicenna. Herbalists today prescribe it to counter depression, stress, insomnia and melancholy. It can help lower high blood pres-sure, and its pleasant lemony smell and taste have made it popular as an everyday tea, or ingredient of wine-cups for centuries. Add its leaves to salads and soups. The freshly-gathered leaves are far more effective than the dried, so grow your own Balm plant.

At times of prolonged stress, try a Balm bath at bedtime, 2 to 3 nights a week, suggest German herbalists Barbara and Peter Theiss. Soak 3 handfuls of the dried herb in cold water overnight, then bring them slowly to the boil; strain and add to your bath. This is particularly useful for children worrying about exams.

Other safe and effective nerve relaxants are **Hops, Lavender, Limeflower, Passion flowers, Peppermint** and **Hyssop**. Drink them as herbal infusions, or add a stronger

infusion of them to a bath or a hot footbath. According to recent statistics, more than 1000 million people worldwide suffer from insom-nia; your GP probably sees at least half-a-dozen cases a day, and every High Street chemist is regularly called on for 'something to help me sleep'. Among the side-effects of the sleep-inducing drugs for which so many pre-scriptions are written daily, are that sense of dazed heaviness on waking, chronic tiredness, depression, and loss of sexual desire. Eventu-ally, they can become addictive. There are, however, numerous herbs which will help give you a night of peaceful sleep.

If over-anxiety, palpitations or a racing heart keep you awake, consult your GP. Pal-pitations can also be triggered by certain foods, such as soy sauce and yeast extract. Replace tea or coffee with sedative and anti-spasmodic **Hawthorn** blossom tea 2 or 3 times a day, and take another cup at bedtime. Add a dessert-spoonful of the flowers or leaves to a cupful of

---

Bawme comforts the heart and driveth away all melancholy and sadness: it makes the heart merry and joyfull and strengtheneth the vitall spirits.
John Gerard: The Herball, 1633

---

boiling water, and infuse for 10 minutes. Add a small shot of whisky to the bedtime cup, and a teaspoon of either **Lime** or **Lavender** honey.

People have been known to be overcome by sleepiness in a **Hop** warehouse, and George III could not sleep without his Hop pillow. This is aromatherapy in action; in fact many of the great nerve-relaxants depend for their effec-tiveness on their essential oils. To make your own Hop pillow, you will need 100g/4oz of the dried Hop cones; make a six-inch square pillow-case of soft cotton, stuff it and sew it up. The pillow is either tucked under your normal pillows, or put alongside it; either way, the relaxing aromas will help keep you sleeping gently all night. Among other aromatic relaxants you could put in the pillow are: **Marjoram; Lavender; Mint; Sweet Woodruff; Angelica**; and **Lemon Verbena**. Dried **Rose** petals, powdered dry **Mint**, and powdered **Cloves** make a spicy, sweet-smelling pillow. In her book *Herbs for Fun* Elizabeth Walker suggests this combination: 25g/1oz Lemon Verbena, 25g/1oz Marjoram, a pinch each of Thyme and Mint.

A warm – but not too hot – bedtime bath is a favourite sleep-inducer for many people. Add 4–5 drops of any of the following essential oils: **Lavender, Clary Sage** or **Neroli**. Put a drop on your pillow as well. Lavender is a gentle strengthening tonic for the nervous system and useful for depression. Put Lavender sachets among the sheets and pillow-cases in your linen cupboard. Clary Sage is profoundly relaxing, especially for the stressed and anxious; do not combine it with alcohol, though, warns aromatherapist Patricia Davis, who has known this give rise to frightful nightmares in her clients. Neroli – made from the blossoms of the bitter Orange – is useful for sleeplessness caused by anxiety.

If you feel too tired for a bath, try a hot footbath; add to it a few drops of any of these oils.

Cowslips are a centuries-old country remedy for insomnia, nervous excitability and hysteric states; and most cottagers kept a store of bright yellow Cowslip syrup on hand for such emergencies.
N.B. Too much can cause dizziness or a 'spaced-out' feeling in some sensitive people.

One of the most effective herbs for the insomnia that results from stress is **Limeflower**, which is popular as a pleasant-tasting tea.
Eat a thick creamy **Lettuce** soup for supper if you have problems sleeping; a famous French recipe is called *Le Potage du Pere Tranquille*. Or make a strong infusion from half-a-dozen of the leaves and drink it at bedtime. Lettuce is a natural soporific.

A GENTLEMAN of good Estate, living near Ivingho in Bucks . . . would gather and dry the (Cowslip) Flowers in the Sun, which he afterwards kept in a Paper-Bag, for making Tea of them, which he did many Nights to make him sleep. Others for this Purpose make a Wine of them.
The Country Housewife's Family Companion
(W. Ellis, 1750)

Depression – even the deepest, blackest kind which seems to be entirely 'in the mind' – can result from nutritional deficiency or food sensitivities. If it descends on you out of the blue, and for no particular reason that you can see, this is especially likely to be the case. The blues can also follow illness – post- 'flu depression is well-known, as is post-natal depression. Even when your depression is caused by events in your life which temporarily overwhelm your spirits, eating the right foods can help restore the strength and vitality you need so badly. Avoid refined carbohydrates – robbed of the B vitamins you badly need; eat **Wholeweat** bread, brown **Rice, Sesame** and **Sunflower** seeds – rich in minerals. Try **Buckwheat** and **Millet**; enjoy black **Grapes**; eat plenty of **Broccoli, Cabbage, Watercress** and **Beetroot**. And cut out all alcohol.

In any nervous problem, it is essential to cut out, or drastically reduce, tea and coffee intake; instead, drink **Rosemary, Lavender, Lime blossom** or **Thyme** tea. **Vervain** is particularly good; it nourishes and fortifies the nervous system, relaxing stress and tension. Put 1-3 tsp of the dried herb in a cupful of boiling water and infuse for 10 minutes. Drink 3 times a day. **Lemon Verbena** is a related herb, with some of the same anti-spasmodic powers. With the exception of Limeflower, all of these teas, however, should be drunk occasionally rather than regularly. Switch from one to another (see Tea-Time, p.47, for more suggestions).

Severe headaches, debility, depression, neuralgia and shingles are all indications that prolonged stress is taking a heavy toll of your vital powers. Herbalists turn to **Oats** for relief, a wonder food for the nervous system. Eat porridge and muesli regularly. Use organically-grown oats, and coarse medium or fine oatmeal.

Headaches are one painful product of nervous tension. Try a tisane of **Rosemary, Balm, Marjoram, Orange blossom** or **Peppermint**. Or try a **Cabbage** compress over your forehead (see p.96). Try adding 6 drops of **Lavender** or Peppermint essential oil to a bowl of icy water, soak in this and wring out a piece of cotton or linen; apply this cold compress to the nape of your neck or your temples. Take a footbath – as hot as you can bear it – to which add a few drops of Lavender oil. You can also make a strong infusion with 5-6 sprigs of Rosemary, and use it for a hot footbath. After either of these, plunge your feet briefly into icy water, then towel and warm them.

Apply a cold **Cider** vinegar compress to your forehead or the back of your neck.

Make extra-strong Chamomile tea and apply a hot compress to your forehead, or the nape of your neck.

Try a Macrobiotic remedy – a Tofu plaster. Take a big chunk – 150-200g/8-10oz of Tofu; wrap it in cheesecloth, then squeeze out the excess moisture. Blend in ½tsp of grated **Ginger**, and enough white flour to make a firm paste. Apply directly to the forehead, and leave on for about half-an-hour.

FEVERFEW FOR MIGRAINES
In the worst headaches this Herb exceeds whatever else is known. . . . A lady of great worth and virtue, the mother of the late Sir William Bowyer told me that having in the younger part of her life a very terrible and almost constant Headache, fixed in one small spot, and raging at all times almost to distraction, she was at length cured by a maid-servant with this Herb.

The British Herbal
(Sir John Hill, 1772)

It is a pity that we lost sight of this invaluable herb for so long! **Feverfew** has now been rediscovered – through the observation of a number of lay people – thoroughly researched, and established as an effective treatment for migraine; even doctors prescribe it today. The dose is the equivalent of a fresh leaf 1-3 times a day.
N.B. Eaten fresh – in a sandwich or salad – it can cause mouth ulcers; if so, take a 125mg capsule 1-3 times a day. (If the capsules seem oddly ineffectual, it could be that they contain very little actual Feverfew; unless you react to the fresh leaves, grow your own.)
Better still, try to find out *why* you keep

getting migraines. Food allergies may be a problem; common 'trigger' foods are cow's milk, egg, chocolate, orange and wheat. The artificial sweeteners used in fruit drinks, 'diet' drinks and squashes are another common trigger. Red wine and cheese are other notorious 'triggers'. Keep an accurate food diary in which you note everything you eat over a period of time, and in another column the incidence and severity of migraine attacks. Then you may be able to identify your own food culprit, if there is one.

Shingles – that aching, itching of blistered nerve endings, often right round the trunk – can be the most painful expression of the lowered immunity caused by prolonged stress. Herbalist Ann Warren-Davis finds **Elderflower** tea uniquely effective for shingles – one of those serendipitous discoveries which have marked the history of herbal medicine. She suggests using a teaspoon of the dried flowers to a cup, filled with boiling water and infused covered for a few minutes. 'Drink it three or four times a day,' she suggests, 'I've known it clear up shingles in a day or two.'

A mix of the tinctures of **Hypericum (St John's Wort)** and **Calendula (Marigold)** can be swabbed gently on the painful zone. Or use this mixture of tinctures added to a little cold water for a cold compress. You could try double-strength infusions of both, mixed, for compresses.

The **Houseleek** is a folk remedy worth trying, if you can get hold of some of the fresh leaves. Peel the thin skin from one side, squeeze out the juice and apply it.

Neat **Cider** vinegar swabbed over the painful area has been known to give relief.

Propolis cream applied to the area, at the same time as a Propolis capsule is taken twice a

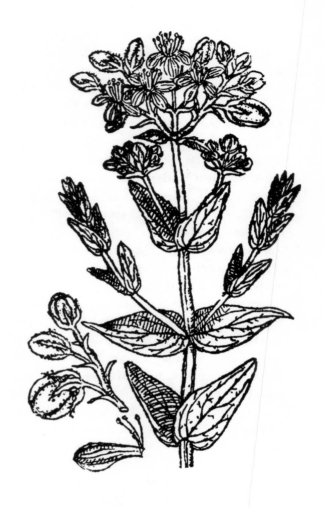

day, has given relief in some cases that have persisted for months.

Aromatherapist Patricia Davis suggests a blend of **Bergamot, Eucalyptus** and **Tea Tree** oils – analgesic and antiviral. If the affected area is small, she suggests painting on a blend of Bergamot and Eucalyptus, neat, with a soft paintbrush, several times a day; or add several drops of each to a couple of tablespoons of vodka. Put a few drops of the same oils in an aromatic bath at night-time. For pain that persists after the blisters have dried up, **Lavender** and **Chamomile** oils can be applied in the same way.

THE RESPIRATORY SYSTEM

If you live in the country and go for a brisk walk every day, you are far less likely to suffer from respiratory problems than people who live in cities, whose lungs are daily assailed by exhaust gases and other pollutants, or who work in factories or offices, or with toxic chemicals.

Pollution is only one threat to the efficiency of your respiratory system, however. Do you breathe properly – through your nose and right down into your lungs? In proper breathing, you can feel the muscles of the stomach wall expand and contract too; this ensures that enough oxygen gets into your lungs – and is thereby circulated via the blood to your whole body.

'Catarrh,' said US Dr Shook, 'is nature's warning signal that a thorough cleansing is needed to assist the faltering eliminative organs.' (See the chapter on Cleansing, p.89).

If you are a smoker, even an ex-smoker, or if you have allergic problems such as asthma, your lungs and respiratory system are likely to be vulnerable, needing lots of tender loving care. Your diet when problems arise needs to be light and cleansing, with plenty of fresh salads and vegetables. A number of foods are particularly helpful – you will find them among the suggestions below. Substitute a herbal infusion for your morning or afternoon cup of tea.

Over the centuries, hundreds of simple herbal or kitchen remedies have been proposed for the problems of the respiratory system – coughs, colds, sore throats, catarrh, mild sinus problems and wheezy chests. The ingredients for most of them will be found in your garden, among your window-sill herbs, in the spice cupboard or the vegetable rack.

Include **Dandelion** and **Nettles** in your diet, cleansing foods which will raise your resistance and vitality. Another Wild Food particularly recommended is freshly picked **Chickweed**, which is almost specific for lungs or any cleansing problems – soothing, healing, nourishing (see Wild Foods, p.42). Vitamin-A-rich **Carrots** should be eaten at almost every meal, grated raw into soups or salads; or drink a small glass of the freshly made juice before meals.

Serious disorders of the lungs and bronchii – asthma, tracheitis, pharyngitis, acute or chronic bronchitis, whooping cough – need professional attention. If your practitioner is a herbalist, he or she will prescribe any of a number of useful herbs she thinks appropriate. There are also mild herbs which will assist rather than counteract the effect of any orthodox drug you may have been prescribed; as a matter of courtesy, though, you should tell your GP what you are taking.

Strong, pungent, cleansing **Horseradish** – like

There were delicious remedies for bad colds. We had linseed tea, a thick liquor made from linseed, flavoured with sticks of black liquorice. We loved to sip this smooth, sweet drink, which was not dissimilar from a cure we gave the cows for colds. No wonder the cattle supped it eagerly! We had thin gruel, sweetened with honey, and hot caudles and treacle possets. In the night we drank blackcurrant tea.

Country Things
(Alison Uttley, 1946)

---

most of the 'hot' herbs and spices – turns up in numbers of country cures for coughs, colds and related problems: for hoarseness, infuse 100g/4oz of the fresh, chopped root in 600ml/1 pint of hot water for 2 hours; then add a little honey. Swallow a teaspoon very slowly; repeat 2 or 3 times.

Nettles are one of the great spring cleaners. In Romany medicine, they are eaten to help rid the lungs and stomach of excess phlegm. For asthma and bronchitis, put a good handful of young Nettles in a pan with 300ml/½ pint of water; bring to the boil and simmer for 5 minutes. Strain and drink the hot juice.

Onions are good for respiratory health in general. For colds, put a thick slice of raw Onion in a cup; pour boiling water over it and let it stand till the water has cooled a little; then strain and drink the water.

There is a red-hot version of this. Simmer ½tsp of **Cayenne** pepper and 2tbsp chopped Onion in a cupful of water for 10 minutes; then strain and drink hot at bedtime.

Hyssop . . . its decoction made of wine and dry figs is good for a cough . . . hyssop water cleans the chest and lungs of heavy phlegmatic humours. It is good for a cough, clears the voice.

Le Livre des Simples

Hyssop is diaphoretic, helps expel excess mucus, and has a soothing, sedative effect. For colds, drink a cupful of a hot infusion 3 times a day. For irritating coughs or bronchitis, combine it with **White Horehound**.

White Horehound has always been one of the most popular country remedies for colds and coughs. The Romans valued it, and seven-teenth-century English housewives found it so indispensable that the first English settlers took plants to North America. Gerard swore by it: 'Syrup made of the greene fresh leaves and sugar is a most singular remedie against the cough and wheezing of the lungs.' White Horehound syrup was a stock item at apothecary shops; it was made into coughs and candy too, and every Receipt Book had an elaborate recipe which included it. An American friend of mine recalls being doctored with her grandmother's famous syrup of Horehound when she had whooping-cough – and very effective it was, too.

This infusion is particularly good for thick coughs with plenty of mucus. Make a hot infusion of White Horehound: 25g/1oz to a 600ml/1 pint; let it stand for 10 minutes, then take a wineglassful. Put the rest in a thermos flask. Take 2-3 more wineglassfuls during the day, and sips of it from time to time when the cough is troublesome.

Mustard footbaths are a good way to nip coughs and colds in the bud – and children enjoy the fuss and the fun of the astonishing bright yellow cure! This is how I made them for our daughters. Take a plastic bucket, put in two heaped tablespoons of ordinary English Mustard powder; half-fill the bucket with water as hot as the victim can stand. Keep a jug of really hot water handy, to top up from time to time. After about 10 minutes, when the feet are bright red, take out and towel them dry. Pull on thick cotton socks and go to bed at once!

Cayenne is one of the great stimulators. Try this formula of the famous US herbalist Dr John Christopher next time you have a cough you cannot shake off: 1 tsp Cayenne powder; 50g/2oz powdered Slippery Elm bark; 1 slice

Lemon; 2tbsp Honey. Infuse in 600ml/1 pint of boiling water; steep and bottle unstrained. Dose: from a teaspoon to a tablespoon, according to age, as often as needed. The Slippery Elm bark supplied by a herbalist, is not to be confused with the Slippery Elm food sold in health-food stores.

This is how to make **Linseed** tea. Thoroughly wash 2tbsp of Linseeds; put them in a pan with 1¼ litres/2 pints cold water, the thinly pared rind of half a Lemon, and a stick of Liquorice. Simmer over the lowest possible heat, covered, for 1½ hours. Strain, add the pressed juice of the Lemon, and a tablespoon of honey. Take a cupful 3-4 times a day. Keep the rest hot in a thermos flask.

The best way to avoid getting a nasty cold is to warm up your system with a hot herbal drink, at the first warning shiver. This will make you sweat a little and stimulate your circulation. Go to bed early, wrap up warmly and have another hot herbal infusion first thing. **Elderflower** and **Yarrow** are both good choices; they are often combined for maximum impact. **Balm** is another good choice.

For the streaming eyes and nose that make life misery during bad colds or in hay-fever, the beautiful little herb **Eyebright** has a drying, anti-inflammatory and near-analgesic effect on the mucous membranes. Make a hot infusion, and take ½ cupful every 2 hours. You can also use the tea – cooled and strained – to soak pads of cotton wool for application to itching reddened eyes.

Cinnamon is warming, stimulating and powerfully antiseptic. Take a dose of it at the first shiver: ½tsp simmered in a cupful of water, with a little honey added to sweeten it. For more about the Cinnamon treatment, see p.37.

TO MAKE A TREACLE POSSET
Boil half a pint of milk. As it rises, add 2 tablespoons of molasses, boil till the curd separates, strain off and boil to serve hot. The lactic acid produced encourages sleep, the treacle acts as a laxative, and the hot drink encourages sweating.

Kitchen Physic
(Dr Fernie)

Drink plenty of **Fenugreek** Tea, which helps dissolve and clear accumulated mucus from the entire body – lungs and respiratory system, intestinal tract, kidneys and blood (see Tea-Time, p.51, for a recipe).

Cabbage leaf poultices are a centuries-old remedy for tight chests, wheezing (see p.00 for how to make them). If it is a cold day, warm them up in a tea-towel on a radiator for a few minutes. Put them on the patient's chest, wrap a thick bandage round them to keep them in place. Leave on overnight.

Drink a small glass of Cabbage juice, sweetened with a little honey. If you do not have a juicer, put 3 or 4 washed and chopped leaves in a food-processor; add a little water, and process. Tip the resulting semi-purée into a pan, bring to the boil, simmer for a couple of minutes, strain and drink.

Elderberries contain viburnic acid, which encourages perspiration; it is useful in coughs, colds, bronchitis and to ward off 'flu. Take 1-2 tablespoons of the Rob (see recipe p.46) in a glass of hot water at bedtime.

Clown's Lungwort was one of the many affectionate names country people used to give **Mullein**, a great remedy for all respiratory problems. It tones the mucous membranes, soothes inflammation, boosts production and expulsion of mucus. In throat or chest infections, try Mullein milk. Put a handful of the big velvety leaves in 600ml/1 pint of milk and bring to the boil; simmer gently for 10 minutes. Strain and drink hot.

Bronchitis and asthma sufferers should avoid milk, however. Instead, make an infusion with a handful of the flowers to a litre/1¾ pints of boiling water; infuse for 10 minutes. Strain through a coffee-filter paper to remove the minute hairs. Drink 3 cups a day, between meals.

DR HAWLEY'S PECTORAL DRINK
Pour a Quart of Barley Water boiling hot
upon an Ounce of Raisins Stoned, a
Quarter of an Ounce of Liquorish and two
figs. Let it stand a Quarter of an hour.
Strain it, give the patient to drink.

The Physick Closet Book
of the Dolben
Family, c. *1785*

Guernsey herbalist Daphne Dunster suggests **Elderflower** tea or syrup to help you cope with the miseries of hay-fever, having tried it herself the first year she developed hay-fever. 'I found noticeable relief from nose blowing within three hours of the first sip,' she says, 'with sniffle production down to about 30 per cent of previous capacity.' (See Tea-Time, p.51, for a recipe.) Drink it hot, a small cup at a time. The rest can be kept in a thermos flask.

Country Living reader Mrs Imogen Nichols, who learned this remedy on one of Daphne Dunster's herbal courses, swears by it. Some years ago she moved into a house now surrounded by Rape fields. When Rape first flowers, Mrs Nichols develops severe 'flu-like symptoms; she then gets out the Elderflower syrup she makes every year and bottles or freezes. She takes 6 small glasses with 1 tbsp of the syrup in hot water, and 2 cups of Elderflower tea, for the first two days, then 2 of each daily while the Rape season lasts. Here is her recipe for Elderflower Syrup.

25 Elderflower heads – shake them free of insects; 500g – just over 1lb – brown sugar; 3 sliced unwaxed Lemons and 2 sliced oranges, both well-scrubbed; 1¾ litres/3 pints water; 50g/2oz tartaric acid. Steep covered for 24 hours, strain into a big pan and bring to the boil; as soon as the sugar is dissolved, remove from the heat. Cool, then bottle or freeze. Imogen Nichols uses pint cream pots.

You can also buy excellent ready-made Elderflower syrups or cordials.

All the members of the **Onion** tribe – which in turn belong to the great **Lily** family – are useful in lung problems. **Garlic** is their undisputed king, useful in coughs, colds, asthma and bronchitis. The easiest and most efficient way to take it is simply to add plenty of it – chopped and raw – to salads. Or you can make it into a syrup, which is very effective against coughs. Slice 3 or 4 large peeled cloves into a little bowl, cover with honey, and leave covered for a few hours. Take teaspoon-doses of the resulting thin syrup every 2 hours or so when symptoms are severe.

A popular Russian treatment for bronchitis is to inhale steam rising from a Garlic infusion. Crush 2-3 cloves into a basin of boiling water, and fill your lungs with the powerful, penetrating healing steam.

For blocked sinuses chop 2-3 cloves of Garlic and leave to infuse in half-a-glassful of cold water overnight. Use as nose-drops. Strong but effective.

In his fascinating collection, *Natural Folk Remedies*, Lelord Kordel describes a study

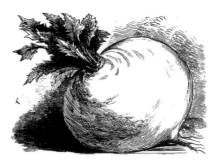

A fourth Receit for Coughs and Asthma – TAKE five or six Figs, as many Cloves of Garlick, and eight or ten Prunes stoned and bruised; infuse all in a Pint of Rum, and fill up if Occasion with another Pint, taking now and then some of it. – The Landlord at the Bear-Inn at Southampton told me nothing exceeds it.
The Country Housewife's
Family Companion
(W. Ellis, 1750)

carried out with army personnel by Dr George D. McGrew of the US Army Medical Corps. Numerous home remedies for hay-fever were tried out, but only one seemed to work – chewing honeycomb caps.

Plantain is very successful in soothing irritated mucous membranes. It contains silicic acid, carotenoids and other chemicals which protect mucous membranes, counter bacterial infections, dissolve mucus and soothe inflammation. Hay-fever sufferers should drink an infusion, hot or cold, 2-3 times a day. Add the young leaves to salads, green vegetables or soups.

To relieve the pain and irritation of sinusitis, try steam inhalations of **Chamomile** or **Yarrow** flowers. Fill a basin with steaming hot water, add a handful of one or the other, and inhale with a towel over your head and the basin. Both flowers contain chemicals called chamazulenes, which are soothing and anti-inflammatory.

Have a cup of hot **Ginger** tea when you come in chilled on a cold winter day. Simmer an inch

of chopped up Ginger root in a mugful of water with a pinch of **Cinnamon** for 20-25 minutes. Strain and drink.

Turnips are a famous old country cure for coughs and colds. Try this cottager's syrup. Hollow out a big Turnip, and fill the cavity with honey or sugar. A syrup will form within 3-4 hours. Take 2 teaspoons from time to time.

Watercress belongs to the same sulphur-rich Nasturtium family; eat plenty of it when you have respiratory problems.

A long peaceful soak in a warm bath can be comforting when you feel full of cold. To make it a therapy as well as a pleasure, mix 4-5 drops of essential oil in a cupful of milk or an unscented shampoo, and add. Choose from **Eucalyptus, Lavender, Hyssop** or **Pine** for coughs and bronchitis; **Rosemary** or **Geranium** to boost your spirits; **Cypress, Cedar** or **Thyme** for a cold.

For a cold: Take a pound of garlick and pound well, adding a quart of wine or good strong old mead, let it macerate well covered, strain, drink lukewarm. The discarded garlick can be used as a poultice for aching joints.
(A thirteenth-century remedy from the famous Welsh herbalist-physicians of Myddvai)

THE SKIN

Skin is amazing stuff. It literally holds us together; keeps foreign bodies out and vital fluids in; helps us stay cool or keep warm; through its myriads of sensory nerve endings, it keeps us in touch with our environment. It is the face we present to the outside world.

The surface of our skin is formed by the two-layered epidermis. The lower layer is a round-the-clock production line turning out millions of new cells every day. Slowly these work their way upwards, becoming flat and horny in the process, until they reach the surface; here they form the protective corneal layer, before sloughing off to become, quite literally, the dust of the biblical phrase.

The dermis below houses nerves, sebaceous glands and sweat glands. Here too are the fibroblast cells which produce collagen, the protein 'glue' which binds the cells together, woven into stretchy sheets. Another protein, elastin, which – as its name suggests – helps preserve the springy resilience of the skin, is also produced here. Interwoven through the entire dermis is a network of tiny blood capillaries which circulate oxygen and nutrients to every cell, carry away wastes and help regulate skin and body temperature.

Without the oil produced by our sebaceous glands even toddlers would have the dry, wrinkled skin of old age; it forms a protective, slightly acidic film – the so-called acid mantle – on the surface of our skin, to trap moisture inside, and protect it from some of the ravages of wind, heat, cold and bacteria.

The operational efficiency of all these protective mechanisms depends on a steady supply of nourishment. Sooner or later, most nutritional deficiencies – particularly those of vitamin A and the B-complex vitamins –

will show up in the skin.

Our skin performs another vital function; it is one of the body's four main organs of elimination. Every day we sweat out around 600ml/1 pint of liquid – more after vigorous exercise. This sweat is not just water; it also contains salt, potassium, and some of the body's wastes in the form of uric acid, urea – waste from the chemical breakdown of protein, ammonia, and lactic acid. Animals injected with sweat actually show symptoms of poisoning.

If your other elimination organs are on a go-slow because of a sluggish liver, overworked kidneys, or chronic constipation, even more of these wastes will be eliminated through the skin; this will produce a sallow, muddy complexion, or a crop of skin problems. If they are the highly toxic wastes of overprocessed junk food, or chemical pollution, then the skin will also be irritated by the poisons passing through it.

Severe nutritional deficiencies will always show up quickly in the skin, since keeping up appearances is low on your body's list of priorities, and nutrients will be shifted elsewhere when badly needed.

Whatever the skin problem, successful treatment must always begin by making sure that diet supplies all the skin's needs, and by dealing with any elimination problems: see the section on Cleansing, p.89. See also the chapter on Skin in 'Beauty Care', p.73, which gives advice on healthy foods to keep your skin in good condition.

Plenty of exercise and fresh air is vital to healthy skin, in addition to a healthy diet. (See What is Healthy Eating? p.22.)

Orthodox medicine has little lasting success

with skin problems, so if you can, consult a professional herbalist to help track down the factors at work in your problem.

TO KILL A FELON QUICKLY
Take a little Rue and Sage, Stamp them
small, put to it Oyl of the white of an Egg
and a little Honey, and lay it to the Sore.
The Queen's Closet Opened
(W. M., 1659)

--------------------o--------------------

There are many herbs which can help restore your skin to health, and keep it in wonderful condition. Some of them will help improve elimination via bowels or kidneys, thereby lightening the load on your skin. Others work to improve local circulation, check bacterial, viral or fungal infection, soothe, heal and prevent scarring. Others tone or nourish. And since the skin can absorb as well as excrete, many of these herbs are used topically, as a wash, salve or compress, as well as being taken internally.

For any skin problem, some of the most effective herbs are also the commonest of weeds: **Burdock; Chickweed; Nettles; Dandelions; Plantain; Yellow Dock**; and **Cleavers**. Burdock is high on the list of herbs to be used, as it soothes and tones the kidneys, eases lymphatic congestion, and helps eliminate excess fat. A useful remedy is equal parts of Dandelion root, Burdock root, and Red Clover – a potent healer and purifier. Take 25g/1oz of this mixture, and simmer for 15 minutes in 750ml/1¼ pints water. Cool, strain and take a wineglassful 3-4 times daily. Use some of it as a wash over spotted skin; allow to dry.

Nettles are another marvellous general remedy; drink a hot infusion – a teaspoon to a cupful – 3 times a day.

Dandelion root is a great friend to the troubled skin; a heaped teaspoon of the root in 250ml/9floz of cold water, left to infuse overnight. In the morning strain, and drink half before breakfast, the rest 30 minutes later.

Heartsease is another wonderful herb for skin problems, eczema, psoriasis and as acne. Dr Henri Leclerc wrote of, ' . . . its usefulness in juvenile acne where, under its influence, one sees the pustules become the site of a flare-up of inflammation, following which they discharge their contents, and fade away leaving no trace'. His suggested dose is: 60g/2¼oz of fresh or dried flowers to a litre/1¾ pints of boiling water; infuse for 10 minutes. Drink 3 cups a day between meals.

Up to 60 per cent of 14–18-year-old girls, and 16–19-year-old boys, suffer the acute misery of acne, when their sebaceous glands go into overdrive and bacterial infection follows. Although GPs often tell their patients that it will clear by their early twenties, nearly a third of those questioned in a recent British survey were still acne victims at the age of 35, and almost 1 in 5 had had it for over 25 years.

Received medical wisdom sees acne as a disease of the sebaceous glands, triggered by the hormonal upheavals of puberty, to be dealt with by prolonged courses – up to 6 months – of antibiotics, or powerful topical applications. Most dermatologists also insist that acne is unaffected by diet.

No herbalist or alternative practitioner would agree with this. 'In my experience,' says US food guru Annemarie Colbin, 'diet has everything to do with acne. Not only did I fix my own bad skin through correct eating, but I have seen among my students a number of severe cases – the large purplish kind of acne on cheeks and chins – *completely cured* within three months by a change of diet.' The most common causes of skin discharge in the form of fatty pimples, acne and boils, are excess fat and protein. In her view, 'if the skin is over-loaded with mucus and/or fat deposits, the kidneys, liver and digestive organs cannot keep up with the disposal work, and the body therefore expels the stuff via the skin.'

If the skin of the acne-sufferer is very greasy, Herbalist Nalda Gosling suggests an infusion of **Lavender**. Pour 500ml/¾ pint of boiling water over a handful of the flowers, leaves and stalks; cover and leave to infuse for 10 minutes. Strain; take a small cup before breakfast and at bedtime. Bathe the skin with the infusion 2-3 times a day.

Drink plenty of beta-carotene-rich **Carrot** juice, and swab spots and pimples with it.

Steam your face 5-10 minutes daily with strong, hot infusions of **Lavender, Yarrow**, or **Chamomile**. Blot dry with tissues; then apply a mix of **Rose** water and **Witch-hazel**.

Drink **Sage** or **Yarrow** tea, and use some of it as a wash. Infusions of **Marigold, Comfrey** leaves or **Chamomile** can also be applied to acne-ridden skin, to soothe, heal and prevent scarring.

Apply **Cucumber** juice every night; re-move it after 10 minutes with **Rose** water.

Treat pimples and pustules with disinfectant **Tea Tree** oil. Dip a cottonwool bud in it and apply 3-4 times a day. Tea Tree oil can pene-trate the skin surface to deal with those ominous bumps which will later ripen into pustules. Caution: experiment on a single pim-ple first – your skin may be sensitive to Tea Tree Oil.

Powerful **Horseradish**, rich in sulphur, is not for the faint-hearted. If you care to try it, grate some of the root and infuse it in hot milk for 30 minutes; then strain and apply the milk to the skin. Or leave a tablespoonful to macer-ate in a cupful of **Cider** vinegar for a week, strain and apply the vinegar.

The dry, scaly, itching skin of eczema affects at least 2 million people in Britain. In hospital trials it has been convincingly linked to food sensitivities, with milk and dairy products, wheat, oranges and chocolate among the com-monest triggers. If your eczema flares up occa-sionally, keep a detailed food diary and try and work out the connections. Stress can be a major factor, as in all problems with an allergic component with bad flare-ups triggered by episodes of severe stress: see The Nervous System, p.108.

Deficiency in essential fatty acids is also a common cause, and oil of **Evening Primrose** is now available on prescription. If this could be the cause of your eczema, persuade your doctor to prescribe it for you, since a course is expensive. Eat oil-rich fish, such as mackerel, sardine, salmon, and extra-virgin Olive oil, fresh hazelnuts and walnuts.

Burdock root, **Nettles, Red Clover** and **Heartsease** – which many herbalists consider specific for eczema – can all be useful in getting to the root of the problem; for doses and pre-paration, see above. **Dandelion**, strongly tonic to the liver, can be specially valuable; see above for preparation and dose. That lowly plant **Chickweed** is a wonderful soother, softener, purifier and healer. Eat plenty of it (see Wild food, p.42), or crush it and apply it fresh to affected skin, binding it in place with gauze. Like Cabbage, it will draw out impur-ities, so change it from time to time.

Herbalist Farida Davidson describes being telephoned by a new patient suffering a severe eczema crisis; she invited her over. 'By the time she arrived, I had a Chickweed bath wait-ing, and this sobbing, burning, itching woman quickly climbed into it. Within seconds the

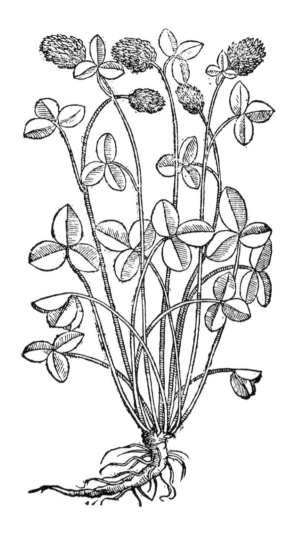

mile; simmer a handful of the flowers in a litre/1¾ pints of water for 10 minutes.

German Chamomile has been used successfully in the treatment of eczema and psoriasis, as well as for very dry, sensitive or inflamed skin.

Make an infusion of either Marigold or Chamomile; let it cool; put it in a plant-mister, and spray it over the affected skin.

Eat plenty of **Watercress**, rich in sulphur and chlorophyll. Nalda Gosling suggests using it as a poultice, too; boil in just enough water to cover, then blend with fine **Oatmeal**, and apply in gauze.

Plantain is another wonderful healer. Wash a handful of the fresh leaves and juice them; if you do not have a juicer, put them in a blender and reduce to a mushy pulp. Apply this to itchy, scaling patches of skin, keeping it in place with a gauze bandage. Or make a plain infusion – 25g/1oz to 500ml/¾ pint of boiling water – strain, cool and use as a lotion.

Aromatherapist Patricia Davis suggests cold compresses with essential oils over areas that are particularly itchy. To make them, fill a basin with cold water – adding a few ice-cubes to make it really cold – then sprinkle 4–5 drops of the oil on the surface. Wring out a clean cloth in the water – a piece of lint, clean old sheeting, or a big cotton handkerchief – picking up as much of the oil as possible, then apply over the area. She has found the essential oil of **Chamomile** most effective, though for some cases **Melissa** is better still (use only 2–3 drops).

Try compresses of a strong decoction of **Sage** – 100g/4oz to 1 litre/1¾ pints of water, simmered for 10 minutes.

heat and the painful itch were relieved. . . .’ Daily Chickweed baths, compresses of Chickweed infusion, a juice fast and systemic treatment for nervous problems completed the cure.

Chickweed oil is another way of applying this soothing plant. Wash a big handful of the fresh plant and blot as dry as possible. Chop it finely, then put in a wide-mouthed jar; cover with Olive oil, and leave to macerate for a week or so. Then strain and rebottle.

When eczema is spread over much of the body, add **Cider** vinegar to your bath, or a strong decoction of **Marigold** or **Chamo-**

Many of the remedies that help with eczema will also be useful in dermatitis. Where hands are affected – by contact dermatitis – it makes sense to wear rubber gloves when using detergents or in contact with well-known triggers. In some cases, heat exacerbates the problem, so try getting someone else to do the washing-up!

Chickweed ointment can be useful to deal with the irritation: Heat 450ml/¾ pint of Olive oil and 50g/2oz of beeswax in a bain-marie; add as much fresh Chickweed – well-washed and dried – as will fit in covered. Leave over a gentle heat for 6-8 hours; then press out the liquid through muslin, and decant into ointment jars. (This is Anne McIntyre's recipe, from *Herbs for Common Ailments*.)

The skin is intimately linked to the nervous system, and psoriasis, like many other skin problems, is often triggered by severe stress or nervous problems. Follow the general suggestions above, and consult The Nervous System, p.108 as well. Herbalist David Hoffmann suggests a tea made of equal parts of Burdock root, Yellow Dock root, Sarsaparilla root and Cleavers. Put 25g/1oz of this mixture in 750ml/1¼ pint water; bring to the boil, and simmer for 10-15 minutes. Strain and drink a wineglassful 3 times a day.

Comfrey, Chickweed and **Marshmallow** ointment can all help with the inflamed or itching skin. Add a strong decoction of **Marigold** to a bath.

Yarrow, according to Nalda Gosling, 'has been found to help clear psoriasis – taken twice-weekly in a warm bath it promotes perspiration and clears impurities through the pores. The herbs are infused for 15 minutes, 1oz/25g to 1 pint/0.5 litre, the liquid added to the bath water, and the herbs in a muslin bag used as a compress and to scrub the patches.'

Cold sores – those irritating little blisters round the mouth – are caused by the same *Herpes* virus that gives you chickenpox; the virus can lie dormant in the system for years, once you have had the disease, to flare up in this form when your resistance is low. If you keep getting them, consult The Nervous System, p.108, for a good nerve-tonic. Meanwhile, those little blisters are very unsightly. Modern research has uncovered an ingenious remedy for them: the sticky residue left in a glass or decanter after almost all the wine has evaporated. It contains concentrated tannins, which do the trick, according to one Canadian scientist.

Or you can use cottonwool buds to paint on any of the following: neat essential oil of **Lavender** or **Tea Tree**; neat **Lemon** juice; or 5 drops each of **Eucalyptus** and Tea tree oil, or Lemon and **Geranium**, added to a tablespoonful of vodka or gin, or ordinary alcohol and then applied carefully to the cold sore.

Boils, abscesses and whitlows on a finger are all signs of lowered immunity or poor elimination. If you are subject to them, follow the suggestions at the beginning of this section. To help bring them to a head, and heal the site afterwards, a number of herbs are helpful.

Try a poultice of boiled **Onions**, applied as hot as you can bear. Or equal parts of **Turmeric** and **Ginger** powder mixed with enough water to make a paste.

Or clean the site carefully then apply 2-3 drops of **Tea Tree** oil, diluted in a teaspoon of any bland oil.
N.B. Some people with sensitive skin react to Tea Tree – go gently at first.
Try powdered **Marshmallow** root or powdered **Slippery Elm**, mixed to a stiff paste with boiling water, and applied hot on a piece of lint, bandaged into place. Renew once or twice a day.

For a whitlow on a finger, put a teaspoon of

tincture of **Calendula (Marigold)** in a small cup filled with water as hot as you can bear; keep the finger plunged in this for several minutes. After just a few applications, the whitlow can be gently squeezed out, and the finger cleaned once more in a fresh tincture-and-water mix; then bandage with Calendula ointment to soothe and heal it.

For more about skin, and how to keep it firm, clear and youthful, see the Chapter on Skin in Part 2, 'Beauty Care', p.73.

Or use a biblical remedy: a Fig baked till it is hot, then applied as hot as you can bear it; keep it in place with a cotton bandage.

'Now Isaias had ordered that they should take a lump of figs and lay it as a plaster upon the wound, and that he should be healed.'

Isaias, xxxviii, v.21

SPECIALLY FOR WOMEN

Women bear children; a series of ingenious anatomical and hormonal arrangements make this possible. Unfortunately, they also render women vulnerable to health problems.

For millions of women these problems – and the discomfort, pain and misery they can bring – have come to be accepted as 'normal'. They are resigned to cramps, irritability, bloating or discomfort bang on cue every month, just as they will expect to be plagued by morning sickness if they become pregnant. And later on, they will wait for the hot flushes, and the depression of the menopause.

But menstruation and menopause, like pregnancy and childbirth, are, of course, completely natural functions. If they are causing discomfort, pain or emotional fragility, don't just put on a brave face or reach for the pills. Instead, give some serious thought to your general health. Any underlying problems will certainly show up as increased discomfort or tension at these times.

A trained practitioner can be of tremendous help. There are a number of herbs: **Chasteberry** *Vitex agnus Castus;* **Wild Yam; False Unicorn Root;** and **Blue Cohosh**, for example, which contain steroidal compounds similar to human sex hormones. These have a tonic, normalizing effect on the reproductive system. For maximum effect, doses need to be fine-tuned for individual women; they are certainly not for amateur home-doctoring. Other herbs can soothe and heal inflamed the mucous membrane, or act as antiseptics. There are also herbs which act as general tonics to the reproductive system; others deal with specific symptoms, such as bloating, cramps and nervous tension.

Aromatherapy, which works on the psyche as well as on a physical level, can also be enormously helpful. Track down a qualified aromatherapist for consultation.

For obvious reasons the contraceptive pill is likely to have a destabilizing effect on the entire reproductive system; if this is the case for you, seriously consider switching to another form of contraception. The Pill is also responsible for lowering levels of at least 3 nutrients – vitamins C and E, and zinc – which will need to be made good. If you are taking the Pill, find a good multi-vitamin and mineral tablet and take it regularly.

In numerous clinical studies and nutritional surveys, menstrual and menopausal problems have been linked with poor eating habits, and with deficiencies in vital nutrients. Too much butter, milk or cheese; too much red meat; too much white flour and white sugar; too much alcohol; an unbalanced diet generally: all of these have been linked with some form of discomfort or pain.

Caffeine, and other alkaloids present in tea and coffee, may be a special threat. ' . . . In any case where hormonal (or emotional) problems appear,' advises British herbalist Simon Mills, 'one should, before doing anything else, simply give up all caffeine for a week at a minimum (and for menstrual troubles at least a month). Then see what one is left with!' Artificial food additives can be a factor, too; period problems have been known to clear up when these were cut out of the diet. Food colourings are prime suspects, as are the artificial sweeteners found in 'diet' drinks, squashes etc.

Check your eating habits (see What Is Healthy Eating? p.22). Particularly vital are plenty of fresh vegetables and the wealth of minerals contained in **Sesame** and **Sunflower** seeds. Make sure, though, that these are fresh when you eat them – the taste will tell you. Sunflower seeds should be pale grey in colour; if they are turning yellowy-brown, throw them away.

Iron deficiency is likely to be a problem for many women, particularly those who have very heavy periods. This is another reason for going easy on the caffeine, since tea and coffee taken at the same meal have been shown to lower the absorption rate for iron and other minerals. As well as meat, fish and eggs, **almonds**, Sunflower and Sesame seeds are all good sources, as are **Watercress, Broccoli** and **Nettles**.

Iron deficiency itself can be a cause of as well as the result of excess menstrual bleeding. In nutritional surveys, women with Pre-Menstrual Syndrome (PMS) problems were often deficient in iron, which helps counter stress amongst its many roles in the body. In one study, 74 out of 83 women stopped having heavy periods when they took 100mg of elemental iron daily. Supplements of vitamin C had much the same effect, probably because this vitamin enhances the absorption of iron. And *all* cases improved with extra vitamin E: 200 international units every other day; vitamin A was found to be valuable too; it is best taken in the form of beta-carotene.

Iron supplements should be taken only as a last resort, when medically advised. Instead, eat iron-rich foods such as meat, fish, dark-green vegetables, Watercress, Dandelion, Nettles and Grapes. Fresh greens and fruit also supply vitamin C to boost iron absorption.

Magnesium deficiency may be responsible for the fluid retention which is a common symptom of PMS. Magnesium is one of the vital nutrients not replaced when wholewheat is refined to produce white flour – only a miserable 15 per cent of it survives. Other good sources are seeds, nuts, and green vegetables.

Cramping pain, caused by spasm or contraction of the muscles of the womb, is one of the most common symptoms of PMS. Any of the following remedies will help. If the pains are liable to come on without warning during the day, when you may be away from home, make up one of the suggested teas; sweeten it with a little honey, and put it in a thermos. Take it to work, where you can drink frequent small sips.

Make **Balm** tea your daily drink, instead of ordinary Tea; fortunately, it is one of the most pleasant of herbal teas to take. (If you really find it impossible to give up your morning cuppa, try 'cutting' it with equal parts of Balm – an old cottagers' trick for economy's sake, when tea was a luxury.)

Another excellent remedy for cramping pain is **Chamomile**; add a tablespoonful to a cupful of boiling water – a particularly high dose; steep for an hour (in a thermos flask, perhaps, to keep it warm), with just a little grated **Ginger** root.

Caraway seeds also help to relieve cramps and nervous tension. Crush 25g/1oz of the seeds, put them in a china jug or basin, pour over 600ml/1 pint of cold water and leave to steep overnight. Take a couple of tablespoons of the strained water whenever you need to.

Cramp Bark, as its name suggests, is another useful remedy. Put 2 teaspoons of the dried bark in a glass or enamel pan; add a cupful of cold water and bring to the boil; simmer gently for 10-15 minutes. You can enhance the effect by adding a little powdered or fresh Ginger root.

St John's Wort is noted for its relaxing effect in nervous tensions and painful cramping. Take it in the form of a tea: 1-2 teaspoons of the dried herb to a cupful of boiling water, infused for 10-15 minutes. Take it 3 times a day, between meals. You could also take it in the form of wine. Macerate a good handful of the fresh flowering tops and leaves in a litre/1¾ pints of good wine for a fortnight; then strain. Take a small glassful as an *aperitif* before the main meal of the day.

Angelica is a warming and stimulating herb, particularly useful for women who feel chilled, low and debilitated during their period, with cramping pain. It will also help sort out menstrual problems generally. Michael Tierra suggests a Tea for such times. 1 part each of Angelica, Cramp Bark, Chamomile; ¼ part Ginger root. Simmer 25g/1oz of this mixture for 15 minutes, covered, in 600ml/1 pint of water. Take ½ cupful, 2-3 times a day.

Warm oil soothed into the lower abdomen, over the womb, can help relax the cramps; use infused oils of **St Johns Wort, Chamomile,** or **Lavender**. Or heat a tablespoonful of **Almond** or other vegetable oil and add 4-5 drops of the essential oil of either Lavender or Chamomile. Otherwise heat up a cupful of water, and add 4 drops of one of these oils; use in a hot compress over your lower stomach, or the small of your back. Cover with a big soft piece of cotton to keep the warmth in for as long as possible, or just lie in bed with a hot water bottle on top of it.

Dandelion is another excellent food-medicine for PMS problems. A good source of iron, it is also one of the best diuretics available, supplying plenty of the potassium which most diuretics leach from the body. Add the young tender leaves to a salad – perhaps the delicious French one on p.43 – or stew it with other green leaves.

The essential oil of **Geranium** can help eliminate excess water. Add 2-3 drops to a morning bath, when its stimulating and anti-depressant qualities will cheer you through the working day.

In the philosophy of Nature Cure, an abnormally heavy menstrual discharge means that your body is suffering from toxic overload, its normal channels of elimination are overwhelmed, and some of the excess is being discharged along with the normal debris of menstruation (see Cleansing, p.89). Cut down on your intake of red meat, cheese, and dairy products if this is high, and eat a variety of fresh vegetables. If the problem persists, consult your GP.

Yarrow tea will soothe menstrual cramps; it has an astringent action, too, which will help check excessive menstrual bleeding. Pour 2 cups of boiling water over a tablespoon of the dried herb, and leave it to steep overnight in a thermos flask. Strain, heat up gently, and drink a cupful first thing in the morning, another last thing at night.

Shepherd's Purse is another useful astringent. Dr Leclerc wrote of it, 'My usage of this plant has proved to me that it is, in effect, a regulator of the menstrual flow . . . particularly active at the two extremes of a woman's life, puberty and menopause, which are so often marked by excess bleeding. . . .' Soak 125g/5oz of the dried plant in 1 litre/1¾ pints of water for 2 hours; then bring to the boil and simmer for 1 minute. Leave to infuse for a further 15 minutes. Take a cupful 3–4 times a day for the 10 days preceding the period.

Women who become tense, nervy and emotionally volatile during the days just before their period have been found to eat increased amounts of dairy products and refined sugar. They are also likely to be deficient in B-complex vitamins and in magnesium. Stress also drains body stocks of B-complex reserves. So make sure that your diet supplies good sources of B-complex vitamins and magnesium, plenty of wholegrains, especially **Oats, Millet** and **Wheatgerm**, fresh nuts and green vegetables – all good sources. Reduce or cut down alcohol and caffeine intake (see The Nervous System, p.108).

Stress, vitamin B deficiency, and a high-intake of saturated fats – as well as the trans-fats found in most margarines and processed polyunsaturated oils and thus in a huge range of ready-made foods – can all contribute to a deficiency in essential fatty acids which help keep the reproductive hormones in balance.

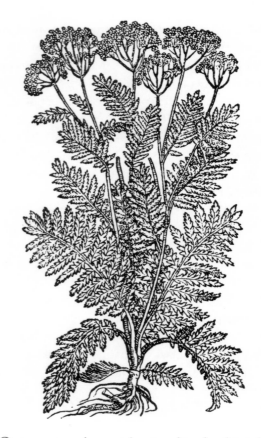

One answer is proving to be the beautiful Evening Primrose, so-called because its lemon-yellow flowers open only in the evening. Oil from the seeds of the Evening Primrose supply gamma-linolenic acid, converted in the body to a substance called prostaglandin PGE1, which seems to help balance hormone activity. In one hospital study, 61 per cent of women trying out Evening Primrose oil for severe PMS were completely relieved of their symptoms. Your doctor should be able to prescribe this for you.

Recurring bouts of nausea can make pregnancy a wretched experience for many women. Recent research suggests that it may be a natural mechanism designed to protect the baby in the womb from toxic substances entering its mother's bloodstream and crossing the placental barrier. This makes sense, since for the first months of its life, the unborn baby has no liver function and no defences of its own.

Surveys of women who suffer from morning sickness often show that their own liver function is defective, possibly due to deficiency in B-complex vitamins; this underlines once more the importance of a good diet, in these months particularly.

If you suffer from regular bouts of nausea, take one of the following simple remedies to help relieve it. But it is important, too, to try and work out just what is causing the nausea; alcohol, nicotine, and the caffeine in tea, coffee and cola drinks are obvious suspects. Eliminate food additives, as far as possible, particularly colouring and artificial sweeteners. Better still, try to avoid processed foods. On mornings when nausea is severe, recall what you ate for dinner the night before, or during the course of the day. If necessary, take extra B-complex.

Chamomile, Peppermint, or **Lime-flower** tea can all be useful; add a touch of grated **Ginger** root to enhance the effect.

Fennel seed tea is excellent for both menstrual and pregnancy problems. Pour 2 cupfuls of boiling water over a teaspoon of the crushed seeds; infuse covered for 10 minutes.

In Macrobiotic teaching, morning sickness is seen as a symptom of excess acidity in the system: if you crave acidic – but alkalizing – fruits such as Lemon or Grapefruit, or sour foods such as sauerkraut, this is almost certainly true for you. Reduce your intake of acid-forming foods such as: white flour (wholegrains are much less acid-forming); white sugar and sugary foods such as cakes, biscuits, and soft drinks. Eat fish rather than meat, fruit and plenty of fresh vegetables. **Umeboshi** plums, sold in health-food stores that stock a Macrobiotic range, are very alkalizing – and very sour! Chew them, or simmer them in

Bancha tea, and sip the tea. Seaweeds are also highly alkalizing.

Chew plenty of fresh **Sesame** seeds, too; they are rich in nutrients vital to pregnant women, and alkalizing mineral salts. Add them to the muesli you soak overnight for breakfast. Instead of plain salt – which may give rise to fluid retention – use gomasio – the salt-and-Sesame mix sold in health stores.

The essential oil of **Orange blossom** or **Neroli** is calming and soothing for the later months of pregnancy; it will also help prevent stretch-marks. Add 4-5 drops to 10ml of **Almond** or **Sunflower** oil, and massage very gently into the skin over your stomach.

Stretch marks themselves are due to sagging connective tissue; eat good wholegrains, organic fruits and vegetables with their skins on (scrub them well), to ensure the vital supply of nutrients, including silicon, which will help keep your skin supple and firm. Vitamin C is equally important, as is the zinc supplied in **Sunflower** and **Sesame** seeds.

Unless you are a sporty and muscular young woman – in which case you might do best to avoid it – **Raspberry** leaf tea is the classic helper for labour, a tonic and stimulant to the whole reproductive system. Take it for the 6 weeks before your baby is due, and you should sail through childbirth. Add 30g/just over 1oz of the dried herb to 550ml/just under 1 pint of boiling water, poured over it; infuse covered for 15 minutes, and drink over the day; sweeten with a little honey, if you like.

Infections of the vagina are very common; according to one study, 72 per cent of young sexually active women suffer from some form of vaginitis. And since the urinary passage in women is vulnerable to infection from the outside, cystitis is far more common in women than in men.

If you notice greater vaginal secretion, or that the discharge is a funny colour or a bit smelly, or feel pain or discomfort, the chances are that you are suffering from vaginitis or inflammation of the vagina. Itching, burning or irritation when you pass water are other symptoms.

N.B. Cases of undue pain or discomfort should be referred to your GP, because if it is caused by an infection, there is a danger that it could spread upwards and lead to worse trouble such as a serious kidney infection, pelvic inflammatory disease or even infertility. Any underlying cause of the problem needs to be sorted out.

Vaginitis can be due to a sexually transmitted infection; it can also be caused by any one of a number of common organisms which lurk around the human frame. It can even occur when the delicate membranes of your vagina become irritated by the chemicals in those deplorable follies, the so-called 'intimate deodorants'.

If you love to loll about for hours in hot bubble-baths, or if you always wear tight-fitting jeans, or nylon tights over nylon pants, or even wear pants to bed, you create the perfect conditions for infectious micro-organisms to flourish (knickers are a very recent invention).

If your doctor pronounces your case of vaginitis a mild one, there is plenty you can do to sort it out. Try to control it without the use of antibiotics: they could exacerbate the sort of fungal overgrowth which may have caused the problem in the first place (see below).

Good hygiene is of the first importance. Wear only cotton pants, and none in bed; if you wear tights, try to find the kind that have a cotton gusset. On a beach holiday do not sit around in wet nylon swimwear; change into another swimsuit, preferably cotton, between

swims. Take only short baths which are not too hot; add 5-6 drops of diluted **Lavender** or

Take Fennel seeds bruised, and boil them well in Barley Water, whereof let wet Nurses and Suckling Women drink very often, in Winter warm, in Summer cold, and let them beware of drinking much strong Beer, Ale or Wine, for they are hot, and great driers-up of Milk, and so are all Spices and to much Salt or salt meat.

The Queen's Closed Opened
(W.M., 1659)

Rosemary essential oil to the bath. If you have a bidet, use it daily to give yourself a good wash; splash a couple of drops of that wonderful antiseptic **Tea Tree** oil into the water. When you use toilet paper, wipe from front to back, or you may be exposing your vulnerable vagina to germs it can do without.

One of the commonest forms of vaginitis is Thrush, caused by the yeast *Candida albicans*; this is a common native of our intestinal tract, but when it proliferates out of control it can cause a wide range of problems. A qualified herbalist can help you with this.

To cope with a case of vaginitis, whatever its cause, your diet should be extra good to enhance your resistance. Sugar encourages *Candida* infestation, even in the form of fruit juices; so does alcohol: cut these out for a few days at least if this is your problem. Eat plenty of **Garlic**, which counters most bacterial, viral *and* fungal infections. You can insert a peeled clove of Garlic into your vagina, wrapped in a little gauze for a powerful local antiseptic effect.

You should not use a douche if you are pregnant, but if you are quite certain you are not, try one of the following:

Douche once or twice a week with 700ml/1 pint of boiled, cooled water to which you have added 2 drops of Lavender, **Myrrh** or **Tea Tree** oil. Patricia Davis suggests diluting the oil in a teaspoon of vodka first. The same solution can be used to soak a tampon; use the kind that come in a thin cardboard cover for easy insertion, or it will at once expand too quickly to use. Leave this tampon in for 4–5 hours, once or twice a week.

N.B. Some people are very sensitive to Tea Tree oil; dab a little neat oil on your skin first, and do not use if it causes any irritation.

Eat plenty of live yogurt, too, and take acidophilus capsules: this will help restore the normal population of micro-organisms in your vagina, which will assist you in overcoming and resisting infection.

Use **Chamomile** or **Thyme** tea in a douche, or to soak a tampon. Either of these herbs can be used – in a strong infusion – in a shallow bath, where you sit for 10 minutes.

Shirley Price suggests sprinkling 6 drops of Tea Tree oil and 2 drops of Myrrh oil into a warm bath. Kneel down in it, and swish the water several times on to the vagina before sitting down in it.

You know when you are suffering from cystitis: the burning pain when you urinate, the frequent urge to do so when there is nothing there – especially at night – and the rank dark urine that often emerges, are all unmistakable signs.

Cystitis is increasingly common among women; if antibiotics were a successful treatment, we should not hear so much about self-help for sufferers. Unfortunately – as with vaginal infections – repeated use of antibiotics often makes matters worse instead of better, and the patient settles down to a dreary routine of infection followed by antibiotic treatment followed by recurring infection.

Professional herbalists can prescribe from a range of highly effective urinary antiseptics; if you are lucky enough to know a good herbalist, seek his or her advice without delay. The sooner treatment is begun, the more effective it is likely to be.

There are a number of remedies, however, that can safely be tried at home.

All the remarks about hygiene in the case of vaginitis (see above p.130) apply with equal force to cystitis, as do the dietary recommendations.

There is one food-medicine which is virtually specific for cystitis: **Cranberry** juice. A substance in Cranberries appear to prevent bacteria adhering to the walls of the urinary tract, where normally they will settle down and start to proliferate. Exposed to Cranberry juice, they lose their grip and get washed away. The same factor may be present in **Bilberries**. If you have a juicer, you can make your own Cranberry juice; take a small glassful twice a day. The Cranberry juice sold in supermarkets, unluckily, is pretty high in sugar – most undesirable in urinary infections. But you can buy raw Cranberries in most supermarkets. If you do not have a juicer, pulp the berries with a little water in a food processor; take a tablespoon twice a day. In one clinical trial, 60 patients with acute urinary tract infections were given 500ml/¾ pint a day, about 3 wineglasses full. More than half of them improved dramatically, and after 6 weeks, 17 patients were completely clear. Add other homely remedies from those suggested here, and you could be one of the lucky ones.

Eat plenty of **Turnips, Celery, Fennel** and **Onions**. Onions are a splendid diuretic, which will help keep things moving in the urinary tract. If you do not like raw Onions, eat Onion soup. Or slice 3-4 Onions into a litre/1¾ pints of hot water, let it stand overnight, and swig during the day.

Cherry stalk tea is an old French country remedy for cystitis, worth trying during the Cherry season. Wash the stalks particularly well; weight out about 40g/just under 2oz of the stalks; let them sit in a litre/1¾ pints of cold water for 12 hours. Then put them in a pan, bring to the boil and simmer for a few minutes. Infuse for 20 minutes, and then strain. Drink 4–5 small cups a day. Or you can pour the hot tea over 225g/9oz of whole cherries (also carefully washed), or Apples sliced into rings; leave to infuse for 20 minutes, then strain, eat the fruit and drink the tea.

Barley water is a centuries-old remedy for irritation and inflammation of the mucous membrane, in whatever part of the body it occurs. Cystitis sufferers should drink plenty of it (see p.99 for how to make it). Drink it un-sweetened.

British herbalist Nalda Gosling, in her excellent book *Successful Herbal Remedies* suggests using **Bearberry** – one of the best urinary antiseptics – in a combination tea, which will exert an antiseptic effect on the walls of the urinary tract in passing. She suggests equal parts of Bearberry, **Horsetail**, a well-known diuretic rich in minerals, and **Marshmallow**, famous for its soothing qualities. Mix them all well, then add a tablespoonful to a big cupful of boiling water; simmer covered for 5 minutes, and allow to cool. Take 2 or 3 times a day.

None of these remedies for cystitis will work for everyone, and they should be used with caution at first.

The menopause does not have to be a pain. There are plenty of women who hardly seem to notice that it is happening. For others, less lucky, it can mean months or even years of discomfort, depression and anxiety – of hot flushes and night sweats, or palpitations or insomnia. They need professional help.

A herbalist can prescribe a number of herbs which can help iron out the problems caused by erratic oestrogen and progesterone activity or their deficiency. The most effective of these are exactly those which most need careful and accurate prescription for individual cases, from a professional.

All the remarks about diet in connection with menstrual problems apply equally to the menopause; cutting out caffeine could be especially useful. To replace it, drink any of the following teas.

Rather charmingly, **Hawthorn blossom** – almost synonymous with spring – bridal **Orange blossom** and **Passion flower** are particularly valued by herbalists for women enduring menopausal problems.

Hawthorn blossom invigorates your heart. It will help calm palpitations, soothe irritability, prevent hot flushes and help you sleep soundly. You can harvest your own Hawthorn blossom in the countryside in May – well away from any agrochemical spraying, please; just give the branches a shake into a paper bag. Or you can buy ready-made teabags. If you use the fresh petals, add a good coffeespoonful to a cupful of boiling water and infuse for 10 minutes. The occasional cupful of Hawthorn tea will not do you much good, however; it needs to be taken regularly over some weeks before its good effects will really be felt. Fortunately, it can safely be taken for a lifetime without ill effect.

Passion flower can help calm the jangling nerves of the menopause. Have 1 cup in the morning, 1 at tea-time, and 1 at bedtime. Add about 40g/just under 2oz to a litre/1¾ pints of water. Heat gently, then boil for a minute. Infuse for 10 minutes.

Orange blossom is another calmer – good for palpitations, spasms and general nerviness. Use a couple of teaspoons to a cupful of boiling water, and infuse for 10 minutes. Drink 2-3 cups a day.

Limeflower is yet another floral aid. It is a great tranquillizer, sedative and anti-spasmodic. Also noted for its cooling effects, it is useful for those suffering from hot flushes. A good pinch should be added to a cupful of boiling water, taken after meals. Or mix Lime blossom and Orange blossom.

All the **Mints** are famous coolers. If you suffer from hot flushes, add plenty of them, finely chopped, to salads; drink **Peppermint** tea; and add a few drops of the essential oil of Peppermint to a bath – not, though, a long hot soak of a bath. Aromatherapist Shirley Price suggests sprinkling a few drops of Peppermint oil on a hanky and inhaling deeply, to help relieve a hot flush; carry a bottle of the oil around with you, to have it to hand when you feel one coming on.

The bright orange petals of the **Marigold** are good for women during the menopause; add them to soups and garnish a salad with them. Use **Balm** freely, too, especially if you suffer from hot flushes, when its cooling qualities will be appreciated; add the fresh leaves with their lemony flavour to soups, salads, green sauces, omelettes or fruit salads.

If night sweats bother you, drink 2 cupfuls of **Sage** tea a day. Put 3 teaspoons of the leaves in a pan, and pour 2 cups of boiling water over them; cover and simmer for 5 minutes. Make this in the morning, put it in a thermos flask, and sip it during the day. Sage is an invigorating tonic, too. You could take it in the form of wine, too; add 75g/3oz of the fresh leaves to a bottle of good red wine and macerate for 10-14 days. This is powerful stuff, though: do not swig it like any old plonk – take a very small liqueur glass of it after dinner.

Nettles, Dandelion, and **Plantain** can all be added to cooked green vegetables or salads, and eaten freely.

Essential oils of **Rosemary** and **Lavender** can be added for stimulating or soothing baths.

—— HERBAL REMEDIES FOR CHILDREN ——

When our daughters were toddlers, I was horrified by how often their small friends seemed to be on courses of antibiotics – often for such relatively minor problems as stomach-ache, coughs or constipation, for which such drugs seemed most inappropriate.

In my experience, most of the run-of-the-mill medical problems of childhood – the snuffles and the sleeplessness, the upset tummies, the mild fevers and the grazed knee – can all be safely and effectively dealt with at home, using mild herbal remedies and a little common sense.

For more complicated problems, such as asthma or eczema, you will need expert help; find an experienced local herbalist who will get to know your children and their constitutions over the years. Of course consult your valued family GP as well.

Children respond to very small doses of herbs, and there are a number of these – ultra-mild, ultra-safe – which are particularly effective for children, toddlers, or babies: **Catnip; Balm; Chamomile; Peppermint; Thyme; Lavender; Marigold**. If you have even a small patch of garden, a balcony, or a patio, it is worth growing them yourself.

When your first baby is still a tiny creature

who sleeps most of the time, it takes a certain amount of courage to administer a herbal remedy instead of calling on the doctor or the chemist. So it is comforting to know that quite often the remedy may not be a dose to be swallowed. A warm compress to relax a tense colicky tummy, a hot footbath, a single drop of essential oil diluted in milk and added to a bedtime bath, or a soothing massage with a little special oil will often do the trick just as effectively. Other medical problems call for true kitchen medicine, a purée of Carrots for mild diarrhoea, perhaps, or Barley water for a feverish child.

Your confidence will grow as your children respond to these gentlest of medicines. Keep a note-book of the remedies you use, and your children's response to them. It is easy to forget, over busy months, what worked for that upset tummy the last time round. For your children, too, it may be a useful record one day. I hope that my generation will re-establish an excellent and age-old custom: that of mothers handing on to their daughters the herbal expertise they've acquired over the years.

N.B. Young children, toddlers and babies do not need and should not be given the same size dose of a herbal remedy as a grown-up. Roughly speaking, if a grown-up dose is a cupful, a 10-year-old will only need a coffee-cupful, a toddler a tablespoonful or two, and a baby a few sips. Alternatively, you can keep a special dropper-bottle (chemists sell these) specially for your baby's herbal remedies; put the chosen infusion into it, and give occasional squirts into the mouth.

Essential oils can be wonderfully effective treatment for a number of childrens' problems, but they are powerful stuff. Never use them undiluted in a baby or toddler's bath, since they could suck their fingers and accidentally ingest them – perilous for a baby gut. Use no more than a drop – usually Lavender or Chamomile – and add it to a couple of tablespoons of milk before you put it in the bath.

ASTHMA

Asthma, like eczema or hay-fever, tends to run in families where there is already a history of such allergy problems. Asthmatic children are often highly-strung, nervy individuals too. They need expert medical attention, and the help of a competent herbalist. But there is also plenty you can do to help strengthen their system, and ease the discomfort and fear of an attack.

Nobody should smoke inside the house. An asthmatic child should sleep in a room with plenty of fresh air, preferably under cotton blankets and sheets rather than a duvet. Plenty of exercise develops sound lungs – swimming is particularly good.

Sensitivity to house dust, mites or chemical pollutants is often a feature. These can never be wholly eliminated, but do your best. And herbs can be useful here – see Herbs Around the House, p.23.

Sensitivity to certain common foods is often important too: milk seems a particularly common problem, particularly as its mucus-building qualities will exacerbate any congestion in the lungs. But if you exclude milk from a child's diet, remember that they still need that protein and calcium from other sources.

Include plenty of **Onions, Leeks** and **Watercress** in the child's diet, green vegetables, including **Cabbage** and lots of fresh fruit. Go easy on the made-up sugary treats such as buns, cakes, biscuits; try and replace white flour and Rice with whole **Wheat**, brown **Rice**; and other grains, particularly **Oats**, which strengthen the nervous system.

Asthma attacks often happen in the night – particularly frightening for children – so make the bedtime bath calming and therapeutic. Add a very strong infusion of **Thyme** which has a soothing, anti-spasmodic effect; or of **Lime-flowers**, which calm the nerves. Otherwise try adding a drop of **Lavender** oil, which is anti-spasmodic and will help – as will the Thyme – if there is any risk of infection.

ALLERGIES

If your child suffered from eczema as a baby, gets lots of colic or a bloated tummy, or has big dark circles under the eyes, or a constantly stuffy nose, suspect an allergy. There are many helpful books written for the parents of children with allergy problems; you'll find them in the Bibliography (see p.156). The important thing to remember is that you can work with your child to develop his resistance and general health; in time he will probably grow out of his allergies, and what seems a huge and endlessly complicated problem now will then be only a minor worry. A good herbalist can be helpful here, prescribing herbs to improve resistance and sort out digestive problems.

BEDWETTING

This can be a cry for help from a lonely or diffident child, a minor irritation of the bladder, or a bit of both. Be very relaxed about it; try not to mention it to any other member of the family if possible, and give the child plenty of reassuring hugs. Avoid sugary foods or lots of drinks late in the evening. Do not give your child cola drinks: their caffeine content can irritate the bladder as well as stressing the nervous system.

Plenty of exercise to improve the circulation is important, and make sure that the child does not get thoroughly chilled, or have wet or cold feet. A calming bath with a drop of **Lavender** oil, or a strong infusion of **Limeflower** will help. So will sips of **St John's Wort** or **Corn**

Silk tea throughout the day; make an ordinary infusion, and give small children a tablespoonful at bedtime. St John's Wort tea is calming and strengthening to the nervous system, Corn Silk is tonic for the kidneys and bladder. **Balm** tea is another great calmer, with a pleasant taste.

If none of this helps, and the problem persists, consult your GP.

BRUISES

A hard fall can produce a painful and badly-discoloured bruise. For mild bruises, swab with diluted tincture of **Arnica**, miraculous stuff, which you can find at a homeopathic chemist; put 2 tsp in a cupful of cold water; or distilled **Witch-Hazel**. If the area hurts badly, apply either of the above in a compress, and keep moist with more Arnica or Witch-Hazel. **Comfrey** oil is also highly effective in reducing bruising.

COLDS, COUGHS, SORE THROATS

Small children catch one cold after another; as long as you deal with them promptly, and don't let them develop into a nasty chest infection, they are in fact a useful muscle-flexing exercise for the developing immune system. Most children enjoy having a day off from school and a little fussing over. And I loved the chance to do a little spoiling, too. . . .

Take action at the first sniffle or shiver. Give the child a cup of hot **Elderflower** and **Peppermint** tea sweetened with honey, keep him warm, and send him to bed early with another small cupful. Keep the bedtime bath short, and add a couple of drops of **Lavender** oil, or a strong infusion of **Thyme** or **Rosemary** to it. With luck that should be the end of the cold. Children love **Linseed** tea as well (see p.115 for instructions).

At night-time, fill a plant-mister with warm

water, add 2 drops each of **Lavender** and **Eucalyptus** and spray it around the room; or if you have an aromatherapy oil burner, leave it in the bedroom till the child is asleep.

A tickly or sore throat means that the virus has taken hold and may develop into a chest infection. Keep the patient home from school, and either in bed or else playing in a warm room. Keep meals as light as possible, with plenty of fresh fruit and green vegetables. Cut out milk and cheese for the time being. Serve raw **Carrot** salads or a purée of very lightly cooked Carrots. **Apples** are especially good; stuffed with Raisins, honey, Almonds, stuck with Cloves: bake them until fluffy, and serve with plenty of **Cinnamon** sprinkled on top. Instead of fruit juice give hot **Blackcurrant** tea; make it by adding hot water to a big dollop of Blackcurrant jam. Or hot **Lemon** and honey.

Get them to gargle – you'll probably have to stand over them while they do this – with either **Sage** tea or **Propolis** (see The Respiratory System, p.115).

A **Mustard** footbath at bedtime is often highly effective (see p.116). The medicinal properties of herbs are very quickly absorbed through the skin of the feet; an old-fashioned remedy for a baby with whooping cough – rubbing the soles of his feet with Garlic – was a quite rational thing to do. So give footbaths with a strong infusion of **Rosemary, Thyme** or **Sage** – all strongly antiseptic herbs.

If the tickle develops into a cough give teaspoon-doses of either **Garlic** or **Turnip** syrup. Make it as follows: take 3–4 fat cloves of Garlic, skin and slice them into a little cup; add a couple of tablespoons of honey, cover and let stand for a couple of hours. Or take a good fresh Turnip, dig out a nice big hole in it and fill it with either honey or brown sugar. In about 2 hours it will have turned into a de-licious, thick Turnipy syrup.

Put a drop of Eucalyptus or Lavender oil on the child's pillow at night.

Make up a massage oil with a tablespoonful of any almond oil and a drop each of Lavender and Eucalyptus; soothe this gently into the child's chest and between the shoulder-blades.

COLIC IN BABIES

For the new mother, severe colic in a baby can be frightening: the tiny fists clenched, the taut belly, the agonized crying. But there are plenty of effective herbal remedies. If it happens rarely, do not worry. If it occurs regularly, try to work out what may be causing it. If you are breastfeeding, it might be something you have eaten or drunk yourself? Alcohol, highly spiced food, Garlic, any of the Brassica family – Cauliflower, Cabbage, Broccoli – too much tea or coffee, too much raw fruit? Or – if there's a tendency to allergy in your own family, indicated by hay-fever, eczema, asthma – the baby could be reacting to common allergens such as Wheat, Oranges and cow's milk in your diet. In the latter case, and if the baby is on formula or first solid foods, it could again be a reaction to one of the commonest allergens – cow's milk, Wheat or Oranges. In this case try a change of diet. For more on this subject, consult the Bibliography, p.156.

Meanwhile, here's how to deal with that colic. Try an infusion of **Chamomile, Dill, Catmint**, or **Balm** tea; ½ tsp of the herbs to a wineglassful of boiling water, infused covered for 5 minutes. Strain, cool and give sips from a teaspoon or from a bottle.

Or simmer ½ tsp of **Angelica** seeds, **Fennel** seeds, **Caraway** seeds or **Aniseeds** in a small cupful of boiling water for 5 minutes, then leave to infuse covered for another 5 minutes; cool, strain and give tiny doses.

Try massaging a little infused oil of **Chamomile** very gently into the baby's tummy. Or soak a piece of lint in any of these teas while they are still warm, and put a compress on the baby's tummy, covering it up warmly, and removing the compress before it cools.

Otherwise add a strong infusion of **Lime-flower**, Chamomile, Balm or **Hops** to the baby's bath.

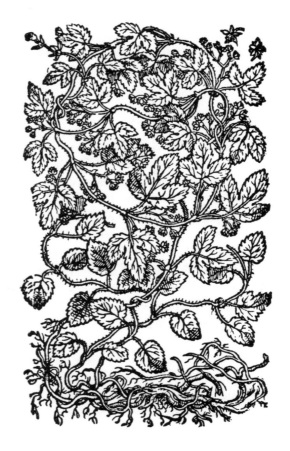

CONSTIPATION

may be due to a food intolerance in a baby who is already weaned. Try eliminating milk or Wheat for a few days; substitute goat's milk and cooked brown **Rice, Oatmeal** or **Millet**. The problem could be too many bland, refined foods in the diet; lots of those little jars are high in modified starch, which may be tricky for a tiny digestive system. Give plenty of puréed, lightly-cooked fresh fruit and vegetables, especially **Carrots** and **Apples**. If it persists, seek professional help.

N.B. Small babies and toddlers should not need laxatives.

CONVALESCENCE

Tackling a viral infection is heavy work for a small person's immune system, and they need plenty of time to rest and recover from it. This does not mean that children should be cosseted and kept under wraps; it does mean giving them a day or two of taking things easy once they are over the worst of a chest infection of feverish cold. Keep them quiet and let them doze or sleep as much as they want to.

Give them plenty of fresh fruit, easily digestible food such as purées of **Carrot** or **Spinach**, light chicken or vegetable and **Barley** soup, and **Arrowroot** or **Slippery Elm** gruels if they look very pale and run-down.

Arrowroot, the powdered root of a plant, is nourishing, easily digested and highly soothing to an irritated digestive tract. It is made into a warm, creamy gruel by adding a cupful of liquid to a teaspoonful of the powder.

The liquid was traditionally milk, but if your child shows any signs of being intolerant or sensitive to this, try **Chamomile** or **Balm** tea instead; use just enough to turn the powder into a smooth paste, then go on adding the rest of the liquid, a little at a time. Whisk to a smooth consistency, sweeten with a little honey, and add a speck of **Cinnamon, Nutmeg** or powdered **Ginger**. Instead of honey, you could simmer a stick of natural **Liquorice** in the liquid you make it up with.

Slippery Elm is soothing and healing for the digestive tract, particularly useful if an illness involved the stomach. Make it just like

Arrowroot, as explained on the previous page. **N.B.** Both Arrowroot and Slippery Elm are sometimes sold ready-mixed with powdered milk. Check the packet if you do not want this.

CUTS, GRAZES, SCRATCHES, SMALL INFECTED WOUNDS

If it is a messy graze, swob gently clean with warm water to which you have added a ½tsp of **Marigold** tincture, or **Tea Tree** oil, in the proportion of 1 part oil to 10 of water. Then use any of the following: Marigold ointment; or a compress with more Tea Tree oil solution; or **Comfrey** ointment; or **St John's Wort** infused oil; or, if you don't have any of these to hand, a **Cabbage** leaf poultice; or plaster it with honey.

When I was a little girl, we were reluctant to display even very nasty cuts or grazes to the grown-ups; out would come the iodine bottle, with its agonizing sting – which might disinfect, but did nothing to stop the pain and smarting, and often left scars behind. The yellow trademark of iodine seems to have been replaced by the red of mercurochrome. Why use either? Any of the remedies mentioned here will not only safely disinfect and hasten healing, but will also soothe away the pain with amazing speed, and prevent scarring.

DIARRHOEA

This is messy in a baby, upsetting in a toddler or child and worrying in either. In a baby it can be caused by sensitivity to milk or Wheat or to Orange juice, or if you are breastfeeding, to something you have eaten yourself (see above, under Colic).

The first step is to stop giving the patient anything to eat that might upset him further, giving his digestive system a chance to rest and right itself once the offending material has been expelled. Give him plenty of fluids, though. Then use kitchen medicine as follows.

For a baby, stop all food and give him only this **Carrot** purée until the diarrhoea has cleared up; 500g/1lb of scraped Carrots sliced and cooked to a purée in a litre/1¾ pints of water; then beat in a blender. Add enough boiling water to make it up to a litre again, finally adding a good pinch of sea salt. Keep it in the fridge, and give over 24 hours. The solids can be given by the spoonful. When the diarrhoea has subsided, give alternate milk and Carrot purée feeds for another day or two. For older children this is also an excellent remedy.

Compresses of warm **Chamomile** or **Ginger** tea can be applied over the child's stomach, or added to a bath.

You could instead make a gruel of brown **Rice** cooked very slowly to a creamy purée in plenty of water, with a little **Cinnamon** bark, or crushed **Caraway** or **Coriander** seeds.

Try a purée of grated raw **Apples**: this can be prepared in a blender, with a little water and a couple of drops of **Lemon** juice, to stop the Apple turning brown. Otherwise try one of the following: plain yogurt; or mashed **Banana**; or **Arrowroot** or **Slippery Elm** (see above, under convalescence); or a very thin purée of **Potatoes**.

If at all possible, the fruit and vegetables given here should be organically grown.

EARACHE
See under First Aid, p.148.

ECZEMA
See remarks under allergies. Your doctor may prescribe corticosteroid creams. These will clear up the excema and stop the itching with gratifying speed, but at a price. Long use will eventually stress your child's immune system, and thin the skin where they are applied. They

do nothing to help resolve the underlying problem. You can tackle this on two fronts: by attempting to identify the cause, and by using common sense, kitchen medicine and herbal remedies to resolve the problem, or soothe and heal the sufferer's skin.

A number of hospital trials suggest that food sensitivities are the commonest triggers, with Milk, Wheat, Oranges and Chocolate as prime dietary suspects; it may, however, be something as improbable as Tomatoes or Peanuts. Keep a food diary for a couple of weeks during which you note every single thing your child eats or drinks (including snacks at friends' houses) and see if they correlate with flare-ups. Then try replacing the problem food temporarily with something else, and see if there is any improvement. Try to build up your child's digestive system and strengthen his resistance, meanwhile, with a first-class diet: plenty of fresh vegetables, fresh fruit, wholegrains with a minimum of sugary treats or high-fat snacks. The suspect foods can be reintroduced gradually once the eczema has cleared, and you may well find that they are no longer a problem. Sound sleep, and plenty of fresh air and exercise are all-important.

A deficiency in certain essential fatty acids may be a cause: ask your doctor to prescribe a course of oil of **Evening Primrose**. This can be absorbed through the skin, so try squeezing the capsules and applying it topically, soothing it gently into the patches of dry, flaky skin. For babies this is often enough to clear the condition. On dry, flaky skin you can use a **Chickweed** ointment, wonderfully soothing for toddlers and older children. Or buy a small jar of aqueous cream from a chemist and add 3-5 drops of the essential oil of **Chamomile** or **Melissa**.

A drop of **Lavender** oil in the bath will help soothe both skin and nerves, as will a strong infusion of Chamomile or **Peppermint**. Or try **Cider Vinegar**; put a spoonful in baby's bath, and half a cupful for older children.

Try making your own infused oil of **St John's Wort** or Chamomile (see p.144), and apply it to itchy, flaky patches of skin. Or apply cold compresses of **Witch-Hazel**, or water to which you have added a teaspoonful of tincture of **Marigold**.

If the eczema persists, consult a qualified herbal practitioner.

FEVERS

These may turn out to be the start of some classic childhood disease such as mumps or measles, or they may be due to some unidentifiable virus. Call a doctor once the child begins to look uncomfortable or the temperature climbs more than half a point or two above normal. Meanwhile, the treatment is bed, rest, very little to eat initially other than simple fruit or vegetable purées, and diluted fruit or vegetable juices, or spring water with fresh **Lemon** juice in it.

On a Spanish family holiday, when Ninka was eight months old, she caught a horrid bug, and was sick, hot and distressed. I took her across the road to a wonderful old Spanish doctor who had eight children of his own. He studied her for a minute, then said simply 'Manzanilla'. This turned out to be Spanish for **Chamomile** tea. I made up a cupful, cooled it and put some in her bottle for her to sip. Within hours she was cool and sleeping peacefully: by the next morning she was her usual happy smiling self again.

Catmint or **Balm** tea are excellent in childish fevers too.

If the fever is high, cool the child by applying compresses to his legs or feet of cool – never cold – water to which you have added a drop of essential oil of **Lavender** or **Pepper-**

mint. The compresses should be removed as soon as they warm up, and renewed. Keep the rest of the child's body lightly covered – do not let him become chilled. To combat infection, use compresses in the same way, but instead of cool water, use a cooled infusion of **Rosemary**.

Put a couple of drops of **Eucalyptus** or **Tea Tree** oil in a plant-mister half filled with warm water, and spray round the room from time to time.

In most of these childhood infections, antibiotics are inappropriate, and many family doctors no longer prescribe them. If your doctor is fairly trigger-happy with the prescription pad, you should think seriously about trying to find another one.

HEADACHES

The temptation to give an instant analgesic to a whimpering child complaining of a headache can be strong, but quite often it is not necessary. Odd headaches that occur for no particular reason can often be tracked back to eating some food with artificial colouring in it, in my own family experience; or a particularly rich meal. Simply sipping warm water will often do the trick, together with a lie-down in a darkened room. A cup of **Chamomile** or **Limeflower** tea can be equally successful, and use some of either of these in a warm compress on the tummy.

For bad headaches, try a cold compress of **Witch-Hazel** on the forehead or the nape of the neck. A little tender loving massage – perhaps with a drop of **Lavender** oil in a teaspoonful of **Almond** oil – around the temples can work very well. Sitting with the feet in a footbath as hot as the child can bear often helps too.

Recurring headaches may very well be due to a food sensitivity; in a trial at Great Ormond St hospital, children suffering from severe and repeated migraine attacks were put on a diet and monitored to identify foods to which they were allergic. When these were removed from their diet for a trial period, 78 of the 88 children completely recovered, 4 greatly improved and only 6 failed to respond. It is usually fairly easy to trace the culprit in such cases; the commonest trigger foods, once more, were: cow's milk; egg; chocolate; Orange, and Wheat, together with the food colouring tartrazine – E102.

HEADLICE

See p.66.

NERVES

Some children seem to be born with a nervous, weepy disposition, easily frightened, often subject to nightmares. A relaxed family atmosphere, and plenty of love and hugs will do more than anything else for them.

Make sure their diet is rich in the nutrients the nervous system needs for its efficient functioning; good wholegrains – **Oats, Millet, Barley** and brown **Rice** as well as **Wheat** – should feature strongly. **Almonds, Sunflower** and **Sesame** seeds are all excellent.

Keep sugar to a minimum, and banish cola drinks from the house: the last thing a nervy child needs is doses of caffeine. By the same token, tea and coffee are quite inappropriate drinks for children.

Limeflower, Peppermint, Balm and **St John's Wort** infusions are all strengthening to the nervous system. Find a combination that your child enjoys drinking; add **Aniseeds, Liquorice** or a little honey for sweetening, and make it a regular morning cuppa. At bedtime give him a Balm bath (see p.143).

If he has difficulty falling asleep, see the section below on Sleeplessness.

NAPPY RASH

Marigold ointment is so effective for tiny inflamed bottoms that you will probably never need to try anything else. Other good remedies are infused oil of **Comfrey, Aloe Vera** gel, or infused oil of **Chamomile**. If you are using disposable nappies, try switching to old-fashioned terry ones for a while – they are not such a chore if you have a washing-machine, and somewhere to hang them. Immediately after changing a nappy, give that sore bottom as much fresh air as possible, rolling on a towel with a rubber sheet underneath it. Nappy rash or not, babies adore to be naked.

SLEEPLESSNESS

There is nothing like rocking for a baby who cannot or will not sleep. If you do not have an old-fashioned rocking cradle – and not many people do, more's the pity – try a little gentle massage. Babies love being stroked. Add a drop of essential oil of **Lavender** to a tablespoonful of bland oil, and gently stroke your baby's tummy, neck, shoulders and spine. A bedtime bath can be soporific: add an infusion of **Balm**, or **Hops**, or **Chamomile** or **Lime-flowers**.

Last thing at night, give little squirts into the baby's mouth of Balm or Chamomile or Lime-flower tea.

In older children, eating too late or too richly can spoil sleep. So can exciting television programmes, or riotous games – 'there'll be tears before bedtime', my husband Henri and I used to say to each other on these occasions.

Make the bedtime bath a time for calming down. Try any of the herbs suggested above for babies. Try a bedtime cup of one of the following – **Chamomile, Limeflowers, Balm, Catnip** or a mixture of two or three, with a little honey added. (Our eldest daughter, Bibi – bright, restless, imaginative, occasionally subject to nightmares – got through gallons of Chamomile tea in her childhood. Perhaps it worked psychologically, too; on a number of occasions, she would come down sleepless to ask for it; by the time I had made it and taken it upstairs for her to drink, she was fast asleep.)

You could try a sleep pillow too. A drop of essential oil of **Marjoram** on an ordinary pillow, or in an aromatherapy burner, can be helpful, too.

SHOCK

A particularly nasty tumble, a gruelling visit to the dentist, bad news, a big emotional upset – any of these can leave children tense, pale and shaken. I always used Dr Bach's Rescue Remedy on these occasions – a few drops on the tongue – and I found that it worked like magic.

TEETHING

Chamomile or **Catnip** tea will both help, in teaspoon doses, or try rubbing a little of either gently into the gums. Chill a Carrot, or a piece of **Marshmallow** root, and let the child chew on it.

WORMS

If your child has a very itchy bottom, looks peaky, or is unusually irritable, restless, tired, has big dark circles under the eyes, or suffers from diarrhoea, constipation or both, suspect worms; they are epidemic in even the most expensive children's schools today. To be sure, look at your child's stools and take a look at his anus an hour or two after he falls asleep; you may see the tiny white threadworms emerging to lay their eggs – a highly disagreeable sight.

However, there is no need to dose your child with the vile-tasting pink stuff your chemist will supply. There are plenty of foods that will eliminate worms just as successfully. They need to be taken first thing in the morning, on an empty stomach, when they will reach the worms with maximum impact, undiluted by friendlier substances. Among foods worms hate are: **Garlic; Onions; Carrots; Cabbage; Lemon**; and **Pumpkin** seeds. The stuff they specially love and thrive on is sugar in any form. Adjust your child's diet accordingly. Try any of the following remedies:

A half-glass of **Carrot** juice taken fasting three mornings running, then repeated a month later; **Cabbage** juice taken the same way.

Pumpkin seeds chewed first thing in the morning; or they can be powdered and mixed with a little water.

In the evening, slice an **Onion** into a glass and cover with warm water. In the morning, bribe the child to drink it.

Throughout the day, include plenty of raw Garlic in salads, and add one or two of these foods unfriendly to worms.

At bedtime, crush a clove of Garlic and add a drop of the juice to a teaspoonful of vaseline ointment. Smear this around the child's anus – a kind of *cordon sanitaire*. A drop of **Lavender** oil diluted in a couple of teaspoons of bland oil will have the same effect.

Check the child's stools to make sure your homely remedies have worked, and repeat a month later.

HOW TO PREPARE HERBAL REMEDIES

The language of herbal medicine can be baffling to the novice, with its talk of tinctures, compresses and liquid extracts. In practise, domestic herbalism calls for a small number of extremely simple techniques. Anything more complicated – infused herbal oils or ointments,

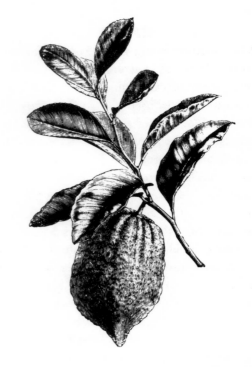

for instance – can almost always be bought from professional herbal suppliers, though you may find it both cheaper and more satisfying to make your own.

Herbs can be successfully extracted by a long soaking in cold water, or in glycerine. Some can be extracted in cold or hot milk, popular in Ayurvedic medicine, where milk is valued for its cooling, soothing qualities. Vinegar is another possibility; in this section you'll find directions for making a number of Herbal Vinegars. The most suitable vehicle for extraction varies from one herb to another, however, and it is difficult to lay down hard and fast rules.

Infusion This is the most commonly used form of domestic herbal remedy. You actually make a herbal infusion every time you pour boiling water into the teapot to make a quick cuppa, and there is not much more to it than that. The chief difference is that a herbal infusion is left for longer, to extract the maximum from its medicinal qualities.

If you are using flowers, leaves, buds and thin stems – the aerial parts of the herb – you take about a teaspoon of dried herb, or 2 teaspoons of fresh, for each cupful of water. Put the herb in a jug or a teapot you keep specially for herbs, and pour the measured amount of boiling water over it. Cover and let stand for 5-10 minutes. Then strain. Keep covered, and once cool store in the refrigerator – for not longer than 48 hours maximum, and preferably no longer than 24 hours.

The infusion can be very gently reheated, but should never be brought to the boil. Otherwise it can be kept warm in a thermos flask. It can be sweetened, if you like, with a little honey.

For colds and chest infections, you can add a stick of natural **Liquorice** to the infusion, for both its sweetening and its soothing properties. For digestive troubles, a few **Aniseeds**, 1 or 2 bruised **Cloves**, or an inch of **Cinnamon** bark can be added to enhance both flavour and activity.

The usual dose is 1 small cupful 3 times a day, between meals, unless otherwise specified.

Decoction Roots, barks and berries need more heat to break down their tough woody consistency and yield up their medicinal properties. So they are simmered in boiling water to make a decoction. Bruise, pound or crush them a little beforehand. Take a teaspoon of the dried root, bark or berries for rather more than a cupful of water – some of the water will evaporate – or 25g/1oz to about 250ml/9floz of cold water. Put both in an enamel or glass pan, bring to the boil and simmer over low heat for 15 minutes. Then strain.

Dose as above, unless otherwise specified.

Tinctures Alcohol extracts the medicinal properties of herbs very successfully; herbalists, who use herbs in great quantity, prescribing them for courses that may last weeks or months, use herbal tinctures, where the herbs are extracted in alcohol. These tinctures keep for a long time, and they are easier to take – small doses in a little water – than a whole cupful of infusion or decoction. However, since they are much more concentrated, working out the correct dosage is trickier; on the whole, they are best left to the professionals.

Herbal Wines Herbal remedies in the form of wines, ales or beers are a tradition almost as old as wine-making and brewing. This is a particularly pleasant way to take medicine.

Hand and Foot Baths As well as being taken by mouth, and absorbed through the digestive tract, much of the medicinal property of herbs can be administered by direct application to the skin. This is a method which has obvious advantages for babies, or when the digestive system is already overburdened. French herbalist Maurice Messegue often administered his herbs in the form of hand or foot baths; the soles of the feet and the palms of the hand are made of particularly porous skin.

To prepare a hand or foot bath, make up a double-strength Infusion or Decoction; pour it into a basin or bucket and fill up with warm water. Soak either your hands as high as your wrists, or your feet as high as your calves. A classic example of this therapy in action is the Mustard Foot Bath (see p.116).

Bath Herbs can also be used in a therapeutic bath; either by adding a few drops of an Essential Oil (see below) or by making a double-strength Infusion or Decoction, and obviously a larger quantity. In this case, the herbs – whether leaves, flowers, root or bark – should be steeped overnight or all day in cold water, then brought to the boil and left to infuse for 10 minutes. Strain them through a sieve, and pour into the already-filled bath. If you're using ready-made teabags, you will need 4 or 5, though 3 would be enough for a small child's bath, and 2 for a baby. **Limeflowers** or **Balm** soothe and relax at bedtime, **Rosemary** gets you going in the morning, **Ginger** works for aches and pains, **Eucalyptus** or **Thyme** for infections; these are all wonderfully therapeutic.

Infused Oil For external use, herbs can also be applied in the form of an infused oil, which is much easier to make than it sounds. It is a wonderfully effective way of applying herbal treatment: **Ginger** for aching muscles; **Chamomile** to soothe pain, nerves or fever; **St John's Wort** or **Marigold** for cuts, grazes and infected sores; **Sage, Rosemary, Thyme** to smoothe into throat or chest to counter infection and **Mullein** flowers for earache.

To make an infused oil, take a good handful of the fresh herb, put in a clean wide-mouthed jar – it should be about a third full – and fill up with a good bland vegetable oil: Almond, Grapeseed, Sunflower or Olive oil (Sesame is good for joint problems, since it is a particularly warming oil). Close up tightly, stand on a sunny window-sill during a good spell of sunshine, and leave for about 2 weeks. Give it a shake from time to time. Then strain through a piece of muslin into a clean jar, and give the muslin a squeeze to get out the last strong drips. As preservative, squeeze in 2-3 capsules of vitamin E, or a little tincture of **Benzoin** – any chemist sells this. Then close up and store in a cool dark place.

Compress Herbs can also be applied in the form of a compress, when you treat a problem locally. Soak a piece of clean lint, gauze or cotton in the herbal infusion of your choice, and apply it to the area to be treated, renewing if necessary.

Steam Inhalations These are a wonderful way to get the soothing, antiseptic and relaxing properties of herbs deep down into stressed, inflamed or congested lungs. Make an Infusion or Decoction of the appropriate herb, add it to a basinful of near-boiling water, drape a towel round your head and the basin to keep the steam in, and inhale very slowly and very deeply for a couple of minutes. Essential oils can be used in this way (see below).

Poultices, Ointment, Creams For the enthusiastic amateur, herbs can also be applied in the form of poultices, ointments, or creams, or administered as syrup. There are excellent books describing these techniques, but in my own busy life, I found there were alternatives involving less fuss or work which seemed just as effective, especially since many of them can be bought ready-made.

Essential Oils Most of the therapeutic powers of aromatic plants are found in their essential oils. Dr Valnet has accurately described these as 'the atomic power of medicine'; it must never be forgotten that they are extremely powerful and highly concentrated substances, each drop representing, perhaps, the therapeutic virtue of many plants. Buy your essential oils from reputable sources; a number of fraudulent or adulterated oils are on sale. In an amateur situation, they should *never* be taken internally. When added to a bath, to oil or to a cream, only the minimum should be used, as even absorbed through the skin their strength will make itself felt. They should always be diluted, either in a carrier oil or – much more simply and effectively – in a little milk, before adding them to your own or a child's bath. This is particularly important in the case of children, who suck their fingers; even a minute amount of neat essential oil, ingested in this way from the surface of the bath, could do great damage to the mouth or sensitive digestive tract.

Most aromatherapists offer a lengthy list of

essential oils which should not be used by pregnant women. Play safe, and use none at all for the first few months; from about the fifth month you can safely use **Lavender, Chamomile** and **Rosemary** in very small amounts.

Essential oils can be used in steam inhalations – see above: you will need 3-4 drops. In a massage oil – add 3-4 drops to 2 tsp of a bland oil. Otherwise you can put a single drop of a sedative oil, such as **Lavender**, on a pillow at nighttime. Or you can put a couple of drops on a hanky, and breathe in from it.

N.B. Essential oils, like all medicines, should be stored safely out of reach of small children.

FIRST AID

In my experience, herbal First Aid wins out over the man-made kind every time. It is cheaper, and you may have it on hand instead of having to rush out and buy it. There are no unpleasant side-effects to worry about, and best of all, it is amazingly effective.

Many of the problems normally covered in First Aid manuals are dealt with elsewhere in this book, in Part 3, 'Remedies'. If your problem is not listed here, look it up in the index.

Some emergencies need immediate medical attention rather than amateur treatment, such as: bad burns; suspected fractures (they should be examined professionally, and may need to be X-rayed, as soon as possible); severe food-poisoning; severe or prolonged diarrhoea; any unusual swelling; any sudden and inexplicable bleeding.

Any kind of poisoning needs urgent attention; keep the telephone number of the nearest Poison Information Centre (your GP will give this to you) somewhere you can find it at once, and ring them if in doubt. If it is obviously poisoning, rush the victim to the nearest hospital emergency department as soon as possible.

At the end of this section, there is a list of the herbal first aid remedies I like to have on hand, as well as a shortlist for travel. Many of the remedies can be bought ready-prepared from chemists, health-food shops or herbal suppliers. (See Useful Addresses at the end of the book for stockists.) Others may be growing in your garden or on your window-sill, sitting in your vegetable-rack, or among your spice-jars.

BRUISES

Bruises from a fall or blow can be very painful. Soothe **Mullein** Oil into the area. Or swab it with tincture of **Marigold**, or with **Witch-Hazel**, or tincture of **Arnica** – homeopathic chemists supply this. If you bruise very easily, consult The Circulatory System, p.92, and eat more fruit and fresh vegetables for their vitamin C content.

Burns In the case of severe burns, summon professional help at once, as the patient will probably need to be treated for shock and dehydration. Meanwhile, the first priority is to cool the burned area as fast as possible, while waiting for help to arrive. Submerge the area of the burn in cold water for at least 10 minutes, or if this is not possible, keep a stream of cold water running over it. If you have it, add 2-3 tsp of tincture of **Marigold** to the water.

Once they have been cooled down, and the worst of the pain has subsided, minor burns and scalds can be effectively treated with herbal remedies. Bear in mind, though, that the risk of infection to badly damaged skin is very high. Apply cold compresses soaked in a lotion of cooled boiled water with 2-3 tsp of Marigold tincture. Or make a **Chamomile** infusion, cool and apply.

Gel from inside the thick greyish-green leaves of the **Aloe Vera** plant has been used for centuries as a folk-cure for burns, cuts and skin problems. Now it is the subject of keen research by dermatologists. One theory is that Aloe Vera can save tissue close to the heart of a bad burn by inhibiting the release of a substance called thromboxane, which seems to be responsible for cell-death and permanent scarring. Aloe also speeds the healing process and stimulates the growth of new tissue.

You can also apply neat essential oil of **Lavender, Comfrey** ointment, or Marigold ointment. **Tea Tree** Oil has a mild analgesic effect which can bring instant relief to a burn or scald; its antiseptic action will prevent infection. Use the neat oil, or a Tea Tree cream for a mild case. **Cabbage** leaves with the central rib removed, dipped in boiling water, crushed with a rolling pin, and then lightly bandaged into place over the area are effective peasant therapy for a burn. Otherwise apply **St John's Wort** oil.

COLDS

There is one moment to stop a cold in its tracks: when you feel the first warning shiver. Act promptly and the cold may never happen. What you need to do is give your circulation a quick boost to raise body temperature, promote perspiration, and with luck, sweat the cold out before it gets dug in. There are a number of tried and tested ways to do this – take your pick. In Greece, according to Jean Palaiseul, they go to bed with a cup of very hot black coffee to which is added the juice of a **Lemon**. Or you can chop up a big **Onion**, put it in a pan with a knob of butter, a little salt, ½

litre of water. Simmer till cooked, add a dash of **Black Pepper** or even **Cayenne** and eat as hot as possible.

Try this Ayurvedic remedy: an inch of fresh **Ginger** root simmered covered in 500ml/¾ pint of water for 10 minutes, sweetened with honey; drink a cupful hot every 2-3 hours. Or simmer 2-3 tbsp of dried Ginger in a litre/1¾ pints of water, add it to a very hot bath, and go straight to bed afterwards with an infusion of **Elderflower** tea – better still, equal parts of Elderflower, **Peppermint** and **Yarrow**. Have a steam inhalation with the essential oil of **Eucalyptus** to stop infection spreading down into your throat and lungs, or use **Benzoin** or **Lavender**.

Take a **Mustard** footbath at bedtime (see The Respiratory System, p.116.) An Elderflower or **Limeflower** footbath is equally good; make a double-strength infusion of either, or both, and add it to the footbath instead of the Mustard. Eat plenty of **Onions, Garlic, Leeks, Carrots.** (See also The Respiratory System, p.115.)

COLD SORES

These are caused by the *Herpes simplex* virus, which lingers in your system if you've ever had chickenpox; they are usually a sign that you are quite run-down. I am indebted to Patricia Davis, in whose useful book *Aromatherapy: an A-Z* I found the only cold-sore remedy that has ever worked for me instantaneously.

Put 6 drops each of the essential oils of **Tea Tree** and **Eucalyptus** in a couple of teaspoons of gin or vodka. Paint the mixture on with a cotton-wool bud at the very first suspicion of that ominous tingle, repeating 3-4 times a day. It will soon dry up, and healing can be helped with a lotion made with a little tincture of **Marigold** or **St John's Wort** in water.

What works for one person does not always work for another, so here are some more suggestions: **Aloe Vera** gel or juice applied neat; **Lavender Oil** applied neat; **Witch-Hazel** combined with tincture of **Myrhh**.

Genital Herpes, the work of a closely-related bug is a case for professional treatment. But if the itching and burning is driving you mad, dab neat **Tea Tree** Oil on the little blisters. You can also add 25–30 drops of the oil to a bath, or add 10–12 drops to 500ml/¾ pint of boiled or purified water, and spray the whole area.

COUGHS

Coughs need to be nipped smartly in the bud, or you'll end up as a nasty case of bronchitis. Steam inhalations with a few drops of essential oils in water not only soothe the irritated mucous membranes but also check any viral or bacterial proliferation. First choice is **Eucalyptus**, closely followed by **Lavender** or **Benzoin**. For a cough remedy very popular in Russia, chop up 2–3 fat cloves of **Garlic**, put them in a cup, add 3–4 tbsp of honey, and leave for a few hours or overnight. Take teaspoon-doses of the thin, odd-tasting syrup every 2–3 hours.

Elecampane root is an invaluable herb in all respiratory problems; a powerful antiseptic that soothes, calms, loosens and helps mucus, it is also a good general tonic for that low, debilitated feeling. It is a useful diuretic, which will help clear infections by boosting elimination. Simmer 10–20g of the root in a litre of water, covered, for 15 minutes: drink 2–3 cups a day, sweetened with honey. Or gargle with warm water to which you have added 4–5 drops of tincture of **Propolis**.

CUTS, WOUNDS, SORES, DIRTY GRAZES

Over the years I must have used kilos of **Mari-**

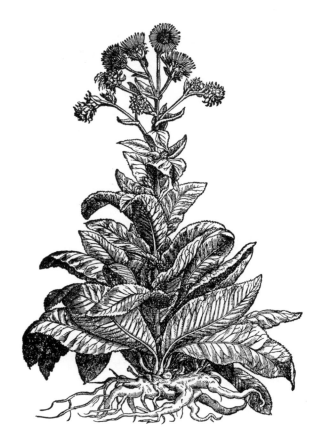

gold **(Calendula)** ointment, which stops pain, disinfects, counters inflammation and speeds healing, as any member of my family can confirm from their own experience. It copes with a dozen different emergencies, including infected pierced ears, paper cuts – which can be extremely painful – knees grazed by a fall, weeping eczema sores on fingers, and the aftermath of boils. Excellent, too, is **Comfrey** ointment, which encourages speedy healing and prevents scarring. **Tea Tree** Oil, which is antiseptic, will not harm tissue or hurt – unlike the iodine we all dreaded as children – and stimulates local circulation to hasten healing. Mildly anaesthetic, it will stop pain.

Afterwards, tape compresses soaked in a solution of Tea Tree and water to the injury. You can also add a few drops of Tea Tree oil to a bland cream, for easier application.

Another useful antiseptic is tincture of **Propolis**.

If you have nothing to put on the wound or graze, apply some honey instead, an old folk-remedy for open sores and infected wounds. Jean Carper tells of a British surgeon who in 1970 announced that he regularly used honey on open wounds after cancer surgery; he found that the wounds healed faster, and had less bacterial colonization than those treated with ordinary antibiotics. In test-tubes, honey killed a wide range of infectious agents.

DIARRHOEA

This is your body's efficient waste-disposal system at work, more of a solution than a problem in most cases. If it is severe, however, or if there is blood in your stools, or if it is accompanied by pain or fever, or lasts more than two days, get professional help. Milder cases such as Spanish Tummy are usually caused by alien bugs in the water supply, abetted by late nights and general riotous living. For remedies, consult The Digestive System, p.99.

Here are some other remedies you might try. Chew Bilberries if you can find them. Drink ordinary tea cold, without milk or sugar; its astringent tannins can help. Chew **Garlic** or swallow Garlic capsules, to counter bacterial infection. Or drink **Cranberry juice**. Simmer 25g/1oz of brown **Rice** – carefully washed – in a litre/1¾ pints of water with 1 teaspoon of salt; for about an hour. Then strain and sip the milky water, a small cupful every 2-3 hours. (See also The Digestive System, p.99).

EARACHE

Earache needs to be treated at the very first twinge, when one of the following remedies should clear it up very quickly: Oil of **Mullein** (see p.144) or the contents of a **Garlic** perle. Sterilize a teaspoon and a dropper in a pan of boiling water, which will heat it up at the same time. Put 4–5 drops of either oil in the teaspoon until the oil is comfortably warm – but not hot – then dropper it into the ear, stoppering the ear with a little cotton wool. Repeat after 3 hours and before bedtime.

US herbalist Brigitte Mars makes her own ear-drops every summer by layering the freshly picked yellow flowers of Mullein in a clean glass jar with slices of Garlic, covering with **Olive** oil. The jar is covered with cheesecloth secured by a rubber band, and left to sit in the sun for 2 weeks. Then she strains and re-bottles the liquid in amber dropper bottles, ready for use. Stored in the fridge, they will keep for up to 2 years. If ear infections are common in your family, make this up and have it to hand. Homeopathic suppliers sometimes stock Mullein oil.

Hot compresses of **Chamomile** tea around the ear will soothe pain and help counter infection. So will a little oil, to which add 1-2 drops of essential oil of **Lavender**, stroked very gently into the area around the ears. Warm the oil first as heat is very soothing for this kind of pain.

If these simple remedies do not work almost immediately and there is already pain and local inflammation, get professional help without delay; serious complications could develop.

If you are holidaying abroad with children, procure the Mullein or Garlic oil beforehand to take with you, because of the risk of infection caught while swimming.

EYES, SORE OR REDDENED

The best first aid is pads of cotton wool soaked in icy-cold **Witch-Hazel**, applied over closed eyes when you are lying down – for at least 5 minutes if possible. Used ordinary teabags work very well, too; if there is a hay-fever victim in the family, get into the habit of saving them in the fridge to cool them. (See also Eyes, p.66.)

FOOD POISONING

See Diarrhoea.

HANGOVERS

The reason why those proprietary fizzy drinks help with the agony of a hangover is because they are alkalizing, and you are in a very acid state 'the morning after'. There are, however, other approaches. Michael van Straten – a naturopath with a kindly view of human frailty – tells me of the **Garlic** cure they resorted to after Bacchanalian orgies in Ancient Rome. Peel all the cloves in a fine fat head of Garlic, and put them in a pan with 300ml/½ pint of red wine. Bring to the boil and simmer for 20 minutes. Strain and share with your hungover partner. This is *not* the hair of the dog: the alcohol goes up in steam; the remaining tannins, plus miracle-working Garlic, do the trick.

A Macrobiotic remedy is to soak an **Umeboshi Plum** – very alkalizing indeed – in hot water or Bancha Tea for 5 minutes. Then sip the water or tea and eat the plum.

An infusion of **Lavender** tops and blossoms can help in a number of ways; it will calm that frightful throbbing, soothe the digestive system, assist the liver to cope, and generally boost the jaded system and the lowered spirits. Oil of **Evening Primrose** is extremely effective at forestalling hangovers if you take 4-6 capsules before you go to bed. Better still, take 4 before you go out, and more at the evening's end. They will not be quite as effective taken the next morning, but will still help undo quite a lot of the damage. Finally, see p.37 for the Jeeves cure!

HEADACHES

There are many causes of a headache. In my experience – almost always in the case of small children – a headache is often the result of a digestive upset, and even sipping warm water slowly will help. **Chamomile, Limeflower** or **Peppermint** tea will be better still.

You may have woken up with it after sleeping in a stuffy room; a brisk walk and a blast of fresh air will blow away this kind. Perhaps you drank too much last night, in which case see Hangovers, above. **Rosemary** tea can help, and so can **Lavender**.

If you have time, soak in a warm bath to which you add either a double-strength infusion of Rosemary or Lavender, or a few drops of the essential oils of either of these, or of **Peppermint**. A very hot footbath often helps, by drawing the blood down from the head; add Rosemary, Lavender or Limeflower tea to it. Ice-cold compresses applied to the forehead or the nape of the neck will help too; add a drop or two of Lavender, Rosemary or Peppermint oil to the water for the compresses.

For headaches following a bad fall or blow, especially if they are exceptionally sharp or severe, or unduly persistent, seek professional advice without delay.

For migraine headaches, see p.113.

HICCUPS

Chew **Dill** seeds, or make a decoction of the seeds and sip it slowly. Very slowly chew and swallow a teaspoonful of sugar. Chew a leaf of **Tarragon**, a useful anti-spasmodic. Try sipping an infusion of **Catnip** tea. Or if you have a friend within reach, sip a teaspoon of neat **Cider** vinegar *very* slowly while keeping your ears stopped.

HOARSENESS

may be the result of a severe sore throat (see

below, p.152) or it may be a problem of voice production. Try **Celery** juice used as a gargle; hold it in contact with your throat for as long as possible. Add 2–3 tbsp of the juice of a glass of hot water and drink 3 times a day.

Try **Carrot** juice the same way. Drink **Thyme** tea; boil a sprig of the herb in a cupful of water for a minute, then take off the heat and leave to infuse covered for 10 minutes. Sweeten with honey, and drink 3 times a day.

In a little book called *The Complete Cider Vinegar* (Thorsons Editorial Board) I found this remedy for a sore throat, which it is claimed can give instant relief in those embarrassing cases when you have to appear in public 'and your voice is hardly above a whisper'. Take 275ml/9floz Cider vinegar; 100g/4oz Honey; 25g/1oz Red Sage; and 15g Self-Heal (see Useful Addresses for stockists). Heat the Cider vinegar with the herbs until it is almost boiling, then remove from the heat and allow to cool slowly. Strain after 24 hours, add the honey, stir till dissolved, bottle and cap securely. Use 2 tsp in half a glass of water. (Self-Heal is quite hard to find, so you may have to try it with just Red Sage.)

INDIGESTION

If you suffer much of the time from indigestion, review your diet and read The Digestive System, p.99.

For an occasional attack, choose from whatever of the following you happen to have on hand. A cup of **Chamomile** tea calms and soothes. **Peppermint** tea relieves cramps, windiness and bloating. **Dill** seeds simmered covered in a cupful of water calms colic; so does an inch of **Cinnamon** bark, simmered covered in a cupful of water for 10 minutes. Sip an infusion of **Rosemary** for gastric pains, an infusion of **Meadowsweet** for heartburn, or

an infusion of **Fennel** to help aid your digestion after a meal.

INFLUENZA

In the early years of this century the **Cinnamon** cure was widely known to doctors as an effective way of nipping an attack of 'flu in the bud. *The British Pharmaceutical Codex* of 1911 lists Cinnamon oil as possessing antiseptic properties, and notes that, 'It is administered on sugar, or as *Spiritus Cinnamonii* for common and influenza colds, and large doses (about 10 minims every two hours) have been found to give relief *within twelve hours* [my italics] in cases of influenza.'

In his book *Kitchen Physic*, published in 1901, Dr Fernie explains the Cinnamon treatment for 'flu and quotes a Dr Ross of Manchester:

In those cases where the Cinnamon treatment has been started within 4–5 hours of the onset of the attack, I have found patients usually able to resume their duties within 48 hours. . . . My experience leads me to believe that no patient, if promptly and systematically treated, need be on the sick list, even after a most severe attack, for more than 5–6 days at the very outside . . . in every case so treated *within 24 hours of the onset*, the patient has returned to his place in society not later than 5 days from the commencement of treatment, and in no case have I been embarrassed by complication of any kind.

The treatment consists of giving 1–2 tsp of a tincture in 2 tbsp of water, or 12ml/½oz of the decoction, every half-hour for 2 hours; then hourly until the temperature returns to normal. The tincture is made by adding 75g/2½oz of bruised Cinnamon bark to a bottle of brandy, and leaving to macerate for a week.

Another version of the Cinnamon treatment is suggested by Dr Valnet. Add half a squeezed Lemon, a tablespoonful of honey, and a large glass of hot water in which a small piece of Cinnamon bark and a Clove have been boiled for 2-3 minutes to a tot of whisky. Leave to infuse for 20 minutes. Like Dr Ross and the BPC, however, Valnet emphasizes that the treatment is effective against colds and 'flu 'as long as it is taken as soon as the first symptoms appear'.

Like colds, an attack of 'flu often begins with a fit of the shivers; if so, follow the suggestions for colds, above. To relieve the dismal aches and odd pains that accompany influenza, take **Boneset** tea. Or simmer 2 tsp of **Fennel** seeds in a cupful of water for 10 minutes and sip. **Ginger, Elderflower, Limeflower** or **Peppermint** teas will all help.

For the sore throat that often accompanies 'flu, see below, p.152.

INSECT BITES AND STINGS
I am one of those luckless people who seem to attract every midge and mosquito in the neighbourhood, while my husband remains unscathed, so I have had plenty of chances to test different insect-bite remedies. Bearing in mind that – as in the case of cold sores – what works for one person does not always for another, here are my findings. The best was one I finally evolved for myself during one particularly troubled holiday.

Plantain, as all the old herbals tell you, is the great anti-poison herb, a wonderful remedy for any kind of bite, sting or poisoning. It is also the commonest of weeds; equally common is **Dock** – and every child knows what Dock can do for nettle stings. So I picked a handful of the youngest, greenest Plantain and Dock leaves, washed and dried them,

chopped them up small, put them in a screw-top jar, filled it up with vodka, and let it macerate a week, giving it a shake from time to time. (Alcohol from the chemist would have been cheaper, but there were none nearby.) Slowly the vodka turned a deep jewel green. It was *very* effective, swabbed on to the stings, as were the crushed leaves rubbed on the stings; if I had had a blender I would have run some through with 2 tbsp of vodka, then added more vodka before putting them in the jar.

Ice-cold **Witch-Hazel** is very soothing when the stinging and burning are at their worst. Neat **Lavender** oil sometimes does the trick. Or add 5 drops each of **Lavender** and **Tea Tree** oil to 1 tbsp of Olive, Sunflower or Almond oil, and soothe into the bite. Tincture of **Feverfew** is said to give instant relief from the pain and swelling of insect or vermin bites. Make this like my Dock and Plantain tincture, above.

According to Dr Vogel, tincture of **Ivy** leaves is good, too. Pick some fresh young leaves, wash them, mince them up or chop them very finely, and let them steep for a week or two in alcohol, then press through a sieve, filter, bottle, and dab on when needed. Or you can try freshly-pressed **Ginger** juice, or rub a slice of **Onion** over the affected area. Crushed **Rue** leaves are said to be very good. So is the juice you squeeze out from the **Houseleek** when you strip the thin membrane off one side of their fat leaves. Tea Tree oil, applied neat, will work wonders for some people. Essential oil of **Geranium** is effective in some cases, using 2-3 drops in a little oil. Tincture of **Marigold** will always soothe and calm. And if you have any **St John's Wort** oil, try that too.

Some people have a very strong reaction to bee and ant stings, and may need medical attention. Treat bee stings – which should be removed – with Onion juice, Lavender oil,

Witch-Hazel, bicarbonate of soda in ice-cold water – immerse the area – Cider vinegar, or the Plantain and Dock tincture, above. Treat wasp stings with Tea Tree oil, Lemon juice, the Dock and Plantain tincture, or Lavender oil.

If you feel really ill after a sting or a number of mosquito bites, as the poison diffuses round your system, the best remedy is an infusion of Plantain leaves; drink 2-3 cups a day.

Of course the best remedy for bites and stings is prevention (see Insect-Repellants, p.13).

NOSE BLEED

Make up a strong infusion of **Yarrow** tea as follows. 2 tsp infused for 10 minutes in a cupful of boiling water and cooled. Soak a piece of cottonwool in the infusion and plug the nose with it. Crush 2-3 **Nettle** leaves, swab up the juice with a piece of cotton wool, and push it very gently up the nostril. Or put a cold **Witch-Hazel** compress over the nose, and another over the nape of the neck. Try soaking cotton wool in freshly-pressed **Lemon** juice and inserting it in the nose. If bleeding persists, or if it happens often, seek professional advice.

POISONS

See note above on Poison Information Centre.

SORE THROAT

The classic remedy for sore throat is **Red Sage**. Make an infusion, strain, add a dash of Cider Vinegar, and gargle for 5 minutes, keeping the liquid in contact with your throat as much as possible. Sip Sage tea, too. **Black-currants** counter infection and inflammation; a spoonful well crushed should be macerated in a cupful of boiling water for 10 minutes. Sip slowly; chew the fruit. **Propolis** has powerful

antiseptic properties, acts as a local anaesthetic, and speeds tissue regeneration; it is particularly noted for its action in the whole mouth and throat area.

SPRAINED OR STRAINED MUSCLES

If the sprained joint becomes very swollen, or if pain does not get better after some treatment, it should be professionally examined to make sure there is no fracture. An ice-pack gives instant relief; Michael van Straten suggests to his patients that they use – and re-use – a bag of frozen peas, carefully marked! Then apply a cotton wool pad soaked in any of the following: neat **Witch-Hazel**; a solution of tincture of **Arnica** or **Marigold** or **St John's Wort**; 2 tsp of any of these in a cupful of very cold water; or an infusion of **Plantain**.

Keep the pad bandaged in place and moisten from time to time with more of the lotion. When the worst of the pain has subsided, try any of the following: 2-3 drops of **Lavender** or **Chamomile** oil in a little bland oil, stroked very gently into the skin. Or apply a poultice of powdered **Comfrey** root mixed to a paste with a little water, or with an infusion of Chamomile; or 2-3 **Cabbage** leaves washed, the central rib removed, gently crushed with a rolling-pin and bandaged into place. These poultices should be firmly but not tightly bandaged into place, and left on for several hours, or overnight.

In India, where **Turmeric** is a popular home remedy, they mix 1 tsp of powdered **Turmeric** with a little honey, smearing it over the sprain twice a day.

A newcomer in this field is **Aloe Vera**, which a number of trainers in the USA are now using to treat a wide range of sports injuries, including sprains, strains and turf burns; they find it penetrates the skin very quickly, reducing inflammation. Increase cell healing time by using Aloe Vera gel in the initial ice-cold compress, soothing more into the injury site 2-3 times a day.

STIFFNESS

If you wake up with a stiff neck or a stiff shoulder **Ginger** is a first-class remedy. Warm a little oil in a pan, then grate a little fresh Ginger root into it, if you have it; otherwise add 1 tsp of powdered Ginger. Leave it in the warm oil for 10 minutes, then soothe into the skin. Or use a little warmed **St John's Wort** oil, or a tablespoon of any bland oil to which is added 6 drops of the essential oil of **Lavender** or **Rosemary**.

SUNBURN

See under burns. But sunburn almost inevitably happens when you are far from home (next time, take a herbal remedy kit with you, see p.00). First of all, *cool* the area. If this means most of you, stand under a cold shower for 10 minutes. This will at least stop the sunburn getting any worse. Get a friend to order some **Chamomile** tea – most Mediterranean bars stock it. Let this cool, and swab the burnt bits with it. Most chemists in France, Italy and Spain sell **Lavender** oil, which is helpful.

TOOTHACHE

Toothache is quite often nothing to do with the tooth: it is the gum that is infected and hurting. Long-term, you need the attention of a good dentist, so make an appointment now.

Meanwhile, here are two remedies, neither of which has ever failed me, or anyone I've suggested them to. Soak a small pad of cotton wool in tincture of **Marigold** and press it to the afflicted tooth or gum. Keep it in place, re-moistening it from time to time, until the aching stops. The lining of your mouth around the swab will probably feel a bit funny, but it will pass, and is nothing to worry about.

Oil of **Cloves** from a chemist is powerful stuff; it is safer and just as effective, in my experience, to let your teeth extract it from a whole Clove. Put it between your teeth at the site of the ache, and keep nibbling gently away at it, until you have chewed it to bits, when you spit out the remains and start on a new Clove, if necessary.

N.B. Use no more than 2 Cloves.

Marigold is antiseptic, soothing to pain, and anti-inflammatory. Cloves are very powerfully antiseptic; indeed, they will also act like a local anaesthetic – dentists in Germany actually use a Clove-based local anaesthetic – so that the pain slowly disappears. Either remedy gets to the root of the problem in every sense of the word, often completely clearing up any infection in either tooth or gum, unlike the traditional aspirin which merely puts you out of your misery for a few hours. But make that appointment all the same.

TRAVEL SICKNESS

See under Nausea, p.00. **Ginger** is so extraordinarily effective against any kind of motion sickness that it is hardly worth mentioning anything else. A convenient way to use it is to make up a small thermos of **Chamomile** tea, using 2 teabags, 2 cupfuls of water, infused for 6 minutes. Strain and pour into the thermos. Grate in an inch or so of fresh Ginger root and close the thermos. Have a small cupful before the journey; take the thermos with you, and if nausea arises, sip another cupful slowly.

THE FAMILY HERBAL MEDICINE CHEST

These are the remedies I like to have on hand. Keep them stored in a clean, cool place, out of reach of small children. Make sure that there are scissors, dropper-bottle, bandaids, packets of sterile absorbent gauze, absorbent lint, gauze swabs, bandages, a clean eye-bath and plenty of hospital-quality cotton wool in the First Aid box.

Tincture of **Marigold**: for burns, toothache, cuts, grazes, boils. Make your own (see p.143) or buy a good ready-made one: sold as tincture of Calendula, the botanical name of Marigold. Weleda make an excellent one, from bio-dynamically-grown plants.

Marigold ointment: for cuts, infected sores, grazes, wounds. Buy it ready-made; again the Weleda ointment is good.

Lavender oil for sleeplessness: put a few drops in the bath; insect bites; burns and scalds.

Garlic perles or **Mullein** oil or the Mullein and Garlic oil described on p.144: for earaches. Prevention or treatment of gut infections.

Oil of **Evening Primrose** in capsules: for PMS, hangovers, and for eczema.

Distilled **Witch-Hazel**: for bruises, sprains, insect bites, reddened itchy eyes – as in hay-fever; relief of mild sunburn. Buy it at any chemist. I keep a big bottle in the fridge.

Tincture of **Propolis**: use as a gargle for sore throats, or to treat painful little ulcers in the mouth or on the tongue.

Essential oil of **Eucalyptus**: for inhalation in colds, coughs, throat or chest infections.

As well as these essential supplies in the medicine chest, I keep the following in stock in my kitchen (for cooking as well as medicine):

Dried herbs for infusions: **Blackberry** or **Bilberry** leaves for diarrhoea. **Chamomile** for mild indigestion, sleeplessness. **Limeflower** for nerves, butterflies in the stomach, sleeplessness. **Elderflower** – combine this with **Peppermint** to take at the start of a cold. If you have space, buy supplies of these loose, and keep them in labelled jars stored out of the light. They are almost all available in teabag form too.

In the spice rack: **Cinnamon** bark – to add to winter drinks, at the start of a cold or 'flu; **Cloves** as emergency treatment for toothache, to add to winter drinks. **Liquorice** root, to add to winter drinks, especially for sore throats.

Fresh or dried herbs: **Sage** for a gargle for a sore throat; **Rosemary** for headaches or low spirits; **Thyme** for an antiseptic tea when colds or 'flu threaten.

In addition: **Onions, Garlic, Carrots, Potatoes. Brown rice. Fresh Ginger root.**

TRAVELLING HERBAL FIRST AID KIT

- **Mullein** oil or **Garlic** perles
- **Marigold** tincture
- **Marigold** ointment
- **Lavender** oil
- A small bottle of **Witch-Hazel**
- Oil of **Evening Primrose**
- Bandaids, pure cotton wool

N.B. When packing Lavender oil or Garlic capsules, seal the jars or bottles up very tightly, and wrap in several layers of plastic bags. (I once packed a leaking bottle of Lavender oil: it took weeks to get rid of the powerful aroma.)

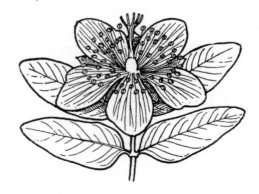

——BOTANICAL NAMES OF HERBS——

Agrimony/*Agrimonia eupatoria*
Allspice/*Pimento officinalis*
Angelica/*Angelica archangelica*
Aniseed/*Pimpinella anisum*
Arnica/*Arnica montana*
Ash/*Fraxinus excelsior*
Avens/*Geum urbanum*

Balm or Lemon Balm/*Melissa officinalis*
Bay/*Laurus nobilis*
Basil/*Ocimum basilicum*
Bayberry/*Myrica cerifera*
Bearberry/*Arcostaphylos uva-ursi*
Benzoin/*Styrax benzoin*
Bergamot/*Citrus aurantium bergamia*
Betony, Wood/*Betonica officinalis*
Bilberry/*Vaccinium mirtillus*
Bistort/*Polygonum bistorta*
Blackberry/*Rubus fruticosus*
Blackcurrant/*Ribes nigrum*
Boneset/*Eupatorium perfoliatum*
Burdock/*Arctium lappa*

Canadian Fleabane/*Erigeron canadense*
Caraway/*Carum carvi*
Cardamom/*Elettaria cardamomum*
Catnip *or* Catmint/*Nepeta cataria*
Cayenne/*Capsicum minimum*
Celery/*Apium graveolens*
Chamomile, German/*Matricaria chamomilla*
Chamomile, Roman/*Anthemis nobilis*
Chervil/*Choerophyllum sativum*
Chickweed/*Stellaria media*
Chives/*Allium schoenoprasum*
Cinnamon/*Cinnamomum zeylanicum*
Cleavers/*Galium aparine*
Clover, Red/*Trifolium pratense*

Clover, White/*Trifolium repens*
Cloves/*Eugenia caryophyllus*
Comfrey/*Symphytum officinale*
Coriander/*Coriandrum sativum*
Cornflower/*Centaurea cyanus*
Corn Silk/*Zea mays*
Cowslip/*Primula veris*
Cramp Bark/*Viburnum opulus*

Dandelion/*Taraxacum officinale*
Devil's Claw/*Harpagophytum procumbens*
Dill/*Anethum graveolens*

Echinacea/*Echinacea angustifolia*
Elderflower/*Sambucus nigra*
Elecampane/*Inula helenium*
Eucalyptus/*Eucalyptus globulus*
Evening primrose/*Oenethera biennis*
Eyebright/*Euphrasia officinalis*

Fennel/*Foeniculum officinale*
Fenugreek/*Trigonella foenum-graecum*
Feverfew/*Tanacetum parthenium*

Garlic/*Allium sativum*
Geranium/*Pelargonium odorantissimum*
Ginger/*Zinziber officinale*
Guaiacum/*Guaiacum officinale*

Hawthorn/*Crataegus oxycantha*
Heartsease/*Viola tricolor*
Hibiscus/*Hibiscus rosa-cinensis*
Hops/*Humulus lupulus*
Horehound, Black/*Ballota nigra*
Horehound, White/*Marrubium vulgare*
Horseradish/*Cochlearia armoracia*
Horsetail/*Equisetum arvense*
Houseleek/*Sempervivum tectorum*
Hyssop/*Hyssopus officinale*

Ivy/*Hedera helix*

Juniper/*Juniperus communis*

Lady's Mantle/*Alchemilla vulgaris*
Lavender/*Lavandula officinalis*
Lemon Verbena/*Lippia citriodora*
Limeflower/*Tilia europea*
Linseed/*Linum usitatissimum*
Liquorice/*Glycyrrhiza glabra*

Maidenhair/*Adiantum capillus-veneris*
Marigold/*Calendula officinalis*
Marjoram, Sweet/*Origanum marjorana*
Marjoram, Wild/*Origanum vulgare*
Marshmallow/*Althaea officinalis*
Meadowsweet/*Filipendula ulmaria*
Mullein/*Verbascum thapsus*
Mustard/*Brassica nigra*
Myrrh/*Commiphora molmol*

Nasturtium/*Tropaeolum majus*
Nettles/*Urtica dioica*
Nutmeg/*Myristica fragrans*

Oats/*Avena sativa*
Origan/*Origanum vulgare*
Orange flower/*Citrus aurantium*

Parsley/*Petroselinum crispum*
Passion flower/*Passiflora incarnata*
Pennyroyal/*Mentha pulegium*
Peppermint/*Mentha piperita*
Plantain/*Plantago major*
Prickly Ash/*Zanthoxylum americanum*
Primrose/*Primula vulgaris*
Purslane/*Portulacca oleracea*

Rose, Red/*Rosa gallica*

Rosemary/*Rosmarinum officinalis*
Rue/*Ruta graveolens*

Sage/*Salvia officinalis*
St John's Wort/*Hypericum perforatum*
Sarsaparilla/*Smilax spp.*
Sassafras/*Sassafras officinale*
Scurvygrass/*Cochlearia officinalis*

Shepherd's Purse/*Capsella bursa-pastoris*
Slippery Elm/*Ulmus fulva*
Southernwood/*Artemisia abrotanum*

Tansy/*Tanacetum vulgare*
Tarragon/*Artemisia dranunculus*
Tea Tree/*Melaleuca alternifolia*
Thyme/*Thymus vulgaris*

Valerian/*Valeriana officinalis*
Vervain/*Verbena officinalis*
Violet/*Viola odorata*

Walnut/*Juglans regia*
Witch-Hazel/*Hamamelis virginiana*
Wormwood/*Artemisia absinthium*

Yarrow/*Achillaea millefolium*
Yellow Dock/*Rumex crispus*

BIBLIOGRAPHY

MANUSCRIPT SOURCES

Collection of Medical, Domestic and Cookery Receipts by Several Hands mid-eighteenth century, Western MSS 4057, Wellcome; Collection of receipts for preserves, cordials, medicine and cookery *c.* 1700, Western MSS 4054, Wellcome; The Dolben family, *The Physicke Closet Book c.*1785, Western MSS 2210, Wellcome; Elizabeth Jacob *Physicall Receipts* 1654, Western MSS 3009, Wellcome; Lady J. Lockwood *Collection of Receipts* 1830–1877, Western MSS 3318, Wellcome; Mrs Jane Parker her Book *Anno* 1651, Western MSS 3769, Wellcome; Madam Bridget Hyde *Her Receipt Book* 1676, Western MSS 2990, Wellcome

GENERAL

Abithel, John Williams ed. *The Physicians of Myddvai,* 1891; A Choice Manuall or Rare and Select Secrets in Physick and Chirurgerie 1693; Anne Hughes: her boke in wiche I write what I doe, when I hav thee tyme, and beginnen wyth this daye, Feb ye 6 1796 Penguin, 1982; *A Book of Fruits and Flowers,* 1653; Bradley, M. *The British Housewife,* 1756; Bradley, R. *The Country Housewife and Lady's Director,* 1676; Cockayne, T.O. *Wort-Cunning and Starcraft of Early England* 2 vols, London, 1864; Digby, Sir Kenelm *The Closet of Sir Kenelm Digby Knight Opened* Philip Lee Warner, 1910; Ellis, W. *The Country Housewife's Family Companion 1750*; A Gentlewoman *The Ladies' Companion, or The Housekeeper's Guide, 1756*; *The Good House-wife's Handbook 1588*; Harington, Sir John *The School of Salernum: the English Version* Humphrey Milford, 1922; Harvey, John *Medieval Gardens* B.T.Batsford, 1981; Heriteau, Jacqueline *Pot-pourris and Other Fragrant Delights* Penguin, 1978; Hertzka, Dr Gottfried, and Strehlow, Dr Wighard *Manuel de la medecine de Ste. Hildegarde, Resiac, Montsurs, France,* 1988; Jarvis, D.C. *Folk Medicine* Pan Books, 1975; McClean, Teresa *Medieval English Gardens 1981;* Markham, Gervase *The English Housewife, 1631;* Middleton, J. *Five Hundred New Receipts, 1734;* Platt, Sir Hugh *Delightes for Ladies, to adorn their Persons, Tables, Closets, and Distillatories, 1609;* Power, Eileen *The Goodman of Paris, 1928;* Smith, E. *The Compleat Housewife, 1747;* van Straten, Michael *The Complete Natural Health Consultant* Ebury Press, 1987; Thompson, Flora *Lark Rise to Candleford* Oxford University Press, 1945; Tusser, T. *Five Hundreth Pointes of Good Husbandrie, 1590*; Uttley, Alison *Country Things* Faber & Faber, 1946; Vasey, Christopher *Manuel de Detoxication,* Editions Jouvence, Genève, 1990; Vogel, Dr H.C.A. *The Nature Doctor* Mainstream Publishing, 1990; W.M. *The Queen's Closet Opened,* 1659–60; Wolley, Hannah *The Accomplish't Lady's Delight in Preserving, Physick, Beautifying and Cookery, 1685*

HERBS AND HERBALS

Bremness, Lesley, ed. *Herbs* Dorling Kindersley, 1990; Buchman, Dian Dincin *Herbal Medicine* The

Herb Society/Rider, 1979; Campion, Kitty *A Woman's Herbal* Ebury Press, 1987; Christopher, Dr John R. *School of Natural Healing* Christopher Publications, Springville, 1976; Culpeper, Nicholas *Culpeper's Complete Herbal* W. Foulsham & Co Ltd; Delmas, Marie *Les Mille Recettes aux Mille Vertus* Magnard-Le Francois, 1990; Fernie, W.T. M.D. *Herbal Simples, 1914;* Frawley, Dr David, and Lad, Dr Vasant *The Yoga of Herbs* Santa Fe, Lotus Press, 1986; Gage, Diane *Aloe Vera* Healing Arts Press, Rochester, Vermont, 1988; Gerard, John *The Herball or Generall Historie of Plantes, 1633;* Gibbons, Euell *Stalking the Healthful Herbs* David McKay Co Inc, New York, 1975; Gosling, Nalda *Successful Herbal Remedies* Thorsons, 1985; Grieve, Mrs M. *A Modern Herbal* Jonathan Cape, 1931; Griggs, Barbara *The Home Herbal* Pan, 1986; Harris, Lloyd J. *The Book of Garlic* Panjandrum Press, San Francisco, 1974; Hoffman, David *The New Holistic Herbal* Longmead, 1990; Kordel, Lelord *Natural Folk Remedies* W H Allen, 1974; Leclerc, Dr Henri *Precis de Phytotherapie* Masson, Paris, 1983; Levy, Juliette de Bairacli *The Illustrated Herbal Handbook for Everyone* Faber & Faber, 1991; Leyel, Mrs C.F. *Elixirs of Life* Faber & Faber, 1948; Leyel, Mrs C.F. *Herbal Delights* Faber & Faber, 1948; Leyel, Mrs C.F. *The Magic of Herbs* Faber & Faber, 1926; McIntyre, Anne *Herbs for Common Ailments* Gaia, 1992; McIntyre, Anne *The Herbal for Mother and Child* Element, 1992; McIntyre, Michael *Herbal Medicine for Everyone* Penguin, 1988; Messegue, Maurice *Maurice Messegue's Way to Natural Health and Beauty* George Allen & Unwin, 1976; Palaiseul, Jean *Grandmother's Secrets* Penguin, 1976; Mills, Simon *Out of the Earth: The Essential Book of Herbal Medicine* Viking, 1991; Opsomer, Carmelia trans. and ed. *Le Livre des Simples* De Schutter, Antwerp, 1984; Rohde, Eleanor Sinclair *A Garden of Herbs* Herbert Jenkins, 1932; Stobart, Tom *Herbs, Spices and Flavourings* Penguin, 1977; Tierra, Lesley *The Herbs of Life* The Crossing Press Freedom, California 1992; Tierra, Michael *Planetary Herbology* Lotus Press Santa Fe, 1988; Tierra, Michael *The Way of Herbs* Unity Press, Santa Cruz, 1980; Tierra, Michael, ed. *American Herbalism* The Crossing Press, Freedom, California, 1992; Treben, Maria *Heath from God's Garden* Thorsons, 1987; Valnet, Dr Jean *Phytotherapie* Maloine, Paris, 1983; Wren, R.C. *Potter's New Cyclopaedia of Botanical Drugs and Preparations* C.W. Daniel, 1988; Griggs, Barbara *Green Pharmacy* Jill Norman and Hobhouse, 1981

FOOD AND COOKERY

Carper, Jean *The Food Pharmacy* Simon & Schuster, New York, 1989; Colbin, Annemarie *Food and Healing* Ballantine Books, New York, 1986; Drummond, J.C. and Wilbraham, Anne *The Englishman's Food* Pimlico, 1991; Edwards, John *The Roman Cookery of Apicius* Rider, 1988; Evelyn, John *Acetaria, 1699;* Fernie, Dr W.T. *Kitchen Physic* John Wright, 1901; Glasse, Hannah *The Art of Cookery made Plain and Easy, 1747;* Greenberg, Sheldon, and Ortiz, Elizabeth Lambert *The Spice of Life* Michael Joseph/Rainbird, 1983; Hartley, Dorothy *Food in England* Futura, 1954; Lamb, Patrick *Royal Cookery, 1716;* Leclerc, Dr Henri *Les Fruits de France* Masson, Paris, 1984; Leclerc, Dr Henri *Les Legumes de France* Masson, Paris, 1984; Leclerc, Dr Henri *Les Epices* Masson, Paris, 1983; Mabey, Richard *Food for Free* Collins, 1989; McNeill, F.Marian *The Scots Kitchen* Blackie & Son Ltd, 1929; Norwak, Mary *The Farmhouse Kitchen* Penguin, 1979; Pegge, Samuel *The Forme of Cury,* 1780; Phillips, Roger *Wild Food* 1983; Raffald, Elizabeth *The Experienced English Housekeeper,* 1805; Spry, Constance *Come into the Garden, Cook* J.M.Dent, 1942; Thorsons Editorial Board *The Complete Cider Vinegar* Thorsons, 1989; Valnet, Dr Jean *Se Soigner par les légumes, les fruits et les cèreales* S.A. Maloine, Paris, 1985; White, Florence *Flowers as Food* Jonathan Cape, 1934; White, Florence *Good Things in England* Jonathan Cape, 1932; White, Florence *Good English Food* Jonathan Cape, 1952; Wilson, C.Anne *Food and Drink in Britain* Constable, 1973

AROMATHERAPY

Davis, Patricia *Aromatherapy: An A-Z* C.W. Daniel, 1988; Drury, Susan *Tea Tree Oil: A Medicine Kit in a Bottle* C.W. Daniel, 1991; Fischer-Rizzi, Susanne *Complete Aromatherapy*

Handbook Sterling, New York, 1990; Lawless, Julia *The Encyclopedia of Essential Oils* Element, Shaftesbury, 1992; Price, Shirley *Aromatherapy for Common Ailments* Gaia, 1991; Price, Shirley *Practical Aromatherapy* Thorsons, 1987; Ryman, Danièle *Aromatherapy* Piatkus, 1991; Tisserand, Maggie *Aromatherapy for Women* Thorsons, 1990; Tisserand, Robert *The Art of Aromatherapy* C.W.Daniel, 1992; Valnet, Dr Jean *The Practice of Aromatherapy* C.W.Daniel, 1980; Worwood, Valerie Ann *The Fragrant Pharmacy* Macmillan, 1990

NATURAL BEAUTY

Buchman, Dian Dincin *Feed your Face*, Duckworth 1973; Lawson, Donna *Mother Nature's Beauty Cupboard* Robert Hale, 1973; Little, Kitty *Kitty Little's Book of Herbal Beauty* Jill Norman, 1980; Messegue, Maurice *Il mio erbario di bellezza* Milano, 1890; Rose, Jeanne *Herbs and Things* Perigee Books, New York, 1972; Rose, Jeanne *Jeanne Rose's Kitchen Cosmetics* Thorsons, 1986

ALLERGY PROBLEMS

Brostoff, Jonathan Dr and Gamlin, Linda *The Complete Guide to Food Allergy and Intolerance* Bloomsbury, 1990; Mansfield, Dr Peter, and Monro, Dr Jean *Chemical Children* Century, 1987; Mumby, Keith, Dr *Allergies . . . What Everyone Should Know* Unwin Paperbacks, 1986

USEFUL ADDRESSES

The Herb Society, P.O. Box 599, London SW11 4RW.

If you are interested in herbs – whether culinary, aromatic or medicinal – then you should join the Herb Society, whose international membership includes professional growers, medical herbalists and gastronomes. They organize lectures and Open Days, and their Quarterly Review is full of useful information for herb-fanciers. Many suppliers offer discounts to members. Send SAE for details.

Rose water, Orange flower water, distilled Witch-Hazel, simple tincture of benzoin, essential oils of Lavender and Peppermint, tincture of Myrrh, and Sweet Almond oil are supplied by many chemists.

Greenscene Indoor Gardens, Burford Lane, Lymm, Cheshire, WA13 0SH. Tel: 0925 75 6328 Greenscene Indoor Gardens supply their Cleanair Plant systems, for both office and domestic use.

To order the cactus *Cereus peruvianus*, send £3.50, to cover postage and packing within the UK, to: **Abbey Brook Cactus Nursery,** Dept. CP., Bakewell Road, Matlock, Derbyshire DE4 2QJ. Tel: 0629 580306

HERBAL SUPPLIES

A number of companies will supply made up pot-pourri, or the dried plant material and refresher oils needed to make your own.

Angela Flanders Aromatics, P.O. Box 2222, London E2 7QB

Angela Flanders makes up a wide range of wonderful pot-pourris to her own recipes, including: Melissa, a tangy and refreshing blend of blue and yellow flowers with a lemony fragrance; and Coromandel, a woody, spicy blend with a Cedarwood base, supplied with refresher oils; or you can order from a range of pot-pourri scenting kits, which come with instructions on how to make up your own. Her shop at 96 Columbia Rd, London E2 7QB is open during the Sunday flower and plant market.

G. Baldwin & Co, 173 Walworth Rd, London SE17 1RW. Tel: 071 703 5550

Huge range of medicinal herbs, roots, barks, powders, gums , balsams, tinctures, including: simple Banzoin, Myrrh, Feverfew, St John's Wort, beeswax, cocoa butter, Mullein and St John's Wort oil, Orange flower and Rose water, Turkey Red oil; and dried flowers for pot-pourri, ready-made mixtures.

The Herbary, Prickwillow, Ely, Cambs CB7 4SJ.
Tel: 0353 88 456
They supply 80 varieties of organically-grown culinary herbs, either freshly-cut of container-grown. Send SAE for their catalogue.

Cheshire Herbs, Fourfields, Forest Road, Little Budworth, Nr Tarporley, Cheshire CW6 9ES. Tel: 0829 760 578
Wide range of herbs – over 180 varieties – herbal vinegars and oils, pot-pourri mixes; their catalogue is a mine of useful information.

Culpeper Ltd, Hadstock Road, Linton, Cambridge CB1 6NJ. Tel: 0223 894054
As well as their pretty little shops up and down the country, Culpeper run a very comprehensive mail-order business. Their enormous range includes: herbal preparations for hair and skin care; bath salts and oils; pot-pourri; pomanders; sleep pillows; herb sachets; soaps; herbal vinegars; fresh herb jellies; and over 170 medicinal herbs. Send SAE for their list.

Mrs Elizabeth Hayes 31 Pyatts Corner, Keevil, Trowbridge,
Wilts BA14 6LY. Tel: 0380 870604
Mrs Hayes makes up a range of Herbal Pillows, 16 different mixes including: pillows for insomnia, migraine and asthma. SAE for list and details.

Barwinnock Herbs, Barrhill, Ayrshire KA26 0RB
Tel: 046 582 338
Organically-grown medicinal, culinary, pot-pourri and dye plants by mail; send 3 first class stams for catalogue.

Neal's Yard Remedies, 3 Golden Cross, Cornmarket St, Oxford OX1 3EU. Tel: 08565 245436
Full range of medicinal herbs, organically grown or wild-crafted where possible; infused oils including St John's Wort and Calendula (Marigold); ointments, including *Stellaria* (Chickweed); essential oils, many of them certified organic by the Soil Association; base oils; flower waters including Chamomile; Orange flower and Rose water; and their own pot-pourri mixes, including blends for the four seasons. Send first-class stamp for catalogue.

Hewthorn Herbs and Wild Flowers, Simkins Farm,
Adbolton Lane, West Bridgford,
Notts NG2 5AS. Tel: 0602 812861
Hewthorn supply 200 native species for woodland, wetland, meadow or your own garden. Their range of decorative, medicinal, aromatic and culinary plants includes lovage, mullein, marshmallow, cowslips and primrose. Send 2 first-class stamps for catalogue.

AROMATHERAPY

The Tisserand Institute, 63 Church Road, Hove, Sussex BN3 2BD. Tel: 0273 206640/772479
Full range of aromatheraphy supplies, including essential oils, massage lotions, bath oils and blended oils. Their Aromastream diffuses vaporized essential oils around a room without heating them. Mail-order catalogue on request.

Bodytreats Limited, 15 Approach Road, Raynes Park, London SW20 8BA. Tel: 081 543 7633
Full-range or organic essential oils, carrier oils, and flower waters, including Damask rose and Orange flower. They also supply amber dropper bottles for your own mixes. Send SAE for detailed price list.

Shirley Price Aromatherapy Ltd, Essentia House, Upper Bond St, Hinckley,
Leics LE10 1RS. Tel: 0455 615466
Essential oils, carrier oils, essential oil distallates including Melissa, Clary Sage and Rosemary water; special essential oil mixes for specific conditions, including herpes/cold sores, insomnia and asthma/hay fever; full range of hair and beauty care preparations based on essential oils.

ORGANICALLY GROWN FOOD

A number of national supermarket chains, including Safeway and Waitrose, now have regular ranges of organically-grown food. If your local supermarket does not, write to the manager and ask why; supermarkets are very sensitive to customer demands.

The Henry Doubleday Research Institute, The National Centre for Organic Gardening, Ryton-on-Dunsmore, Coventry CV8 3LG. Tel: 0203 303517 This is the biggest – and fastest-growing organic movement in Europe. Set in the Warwickshire countryside, it has an organic show-garden, a shop selling a huge range of organic produce, from cheese to vegetables to wine, and an organic-only restaurant that is featured in *The Good Food Guide*. They also organize an annual National Organic Food and Wine Fair. If you would like to go organic in your own garden, they will help with advice and information.

The Soil Association, 86 Colston Street, Bristol BS1 5BB. Tel: 0272 299666 Nearly 50 years old, this pioneering Association actively campaigns for organic agriculture, and acts as a consumer watchdog on food quality issues. Membership brings you their excellent magazine, information, etc. If you are trying to find a local organic food supplier, their Regional List (£2.50 including p&p) gives names, addresses and telephone numbers of farmers and suppliers in your area. Their *Organic Directory Year Book* (£7.95 plus £1 p&p) includes addresses of shops, wholesalers, markets, bed-and-breakfasts, and more.

Pollution-free seaweed Look for the 'Clearspring' label in health-food shops; as far as possible, their range of seaweeds are farmed in unpolluted stretches of sea.

Bottled juices from organically-grown fruit and vegetables The Swiss Biotta range includes: Potato, Carrot, Celery and Beetroot juices, preserved with a tiny amount of health-giving lacto-fermented whey. On sale in most good health-food shops.

PRACTITIONER ORGANISATIONS

The National Institute of Medical Herbalists, 9 Palace Gate, Exeter, Devon EX1 1JA. Tel: 0392 426 022 The leading organisation of qualified herbal practitioners: members undergo four years of training. Look for the initials MNIMH in your local *Yellow Pages*, or send a large SAE for an up-to-date list of members.

The Internation Federation of Aromatherapists, Department of Continuing Education, Royal Masonic Hospital, Ravenscourt Park, London W6 0TN. The leading organisation of trained aromatherapists. Send a large SAE for a list of members, details of training courses, newsletter, lectures etc.

Institute for Complementary Medicine, P.O. Box 194, London SE16 1QZ. Tel: 071 237 5165 The Institute campaigns actively for standards of practice, training, registration and accreditation of complementary therapists. Send a large SAE for information – on qualified therapists in your area, for instance; specify the information you require.

INDEX